The FAT BOY'S downfall

Books by Elmer Wheeler . . .

THE FAT BOY'S BOOK

HOW TO SELL YOURSELF TO OTHERS

TESTED DIRECT SELLING

TESTED RETAIL SELLING

SIZZLEMANSHIP

WORD MAGIC

TESTED PUBLIC SPEAKING

TESTED SENTENCES THAT SELL

The FAT BOY'S downfall

And How Elmer Learned To Keep It Off

BY...
ELMER WHEELER

ILLUSTRATED BY...
Vic Herman

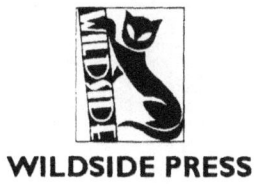

WILDSIDE PRESS

dedicated to

FORLORN FATTIES

who successfully reduced
then bragged . . . .
relaxed . . .
and gained it all back again!

Contents...

1	Elmer the Calorie Hero	1
2	A Great Man's Critics	9
3	The Hindwriting on Elmer's Breadbasket	19
4	Elmer Returns to His Doc	29
5	Elmer Rises Out of the Ashes	40
6	Elmer Organizes the F.B.I. (fat boy's institute)	50
7	The Fat Boy's Thermometer Is Created	60
8	Some Startling Bulge-Banishing Facts	69
9	Even the Small Fry Tell Elmer Off	78
10	How Elmer Spots an F.B.I. Recruit	87
11	Calorie Loses Fat Boy	96
12	Little Known Facts on Fat Boys	105
13	The Fat Boy's Gymnasium	112
14	Don't Shoot the Cook— She's Your Best Friend	121
15	Fat Boys Can Eat Desserts	130
16	Elmer Answers His Mailbag	140
17	The Fat Boy's Kitchen	147
18	My Life with Girth, *by Beth Wheeler*	158
	What's Your "Health I.Q."?	165
	How to Kill the Kalorie in the Kitchen	167

The Fat Boy's Lament...

He pulls up his bay window, sticks out his chins, and makes up his mind to go on a bulge-banishing binge. His wife, best girl, doc, or insurance agent got him started.

Maybe it was the redhead next door.

Anyhow, he takes the Calorie Cure. Sheds off 10, 15, maybe 100 lbs. of high-grade suet—worth 10¢ a lb. in the store, but on him about $100 a lb.

Then he struts for a month, maybe two—maybe six. He takes pride in putting three fingers inside his "horse collar" and pulling out a yard or two of belt.

Then the novelty wears off. He begins to backslide. First —a little on a boat trip or a series of banquets, maybe on vacation or during the holidays.

Nothing much to start with. . . . Then, suddenly, down he shoots on the toboggan slide! He's a fallen fat boy. His downfall is almost pathetic.

That's what happened to Elmer. But then, being the self-elected fat boy's friend, he felt obliged to do something about it—something every fallen fat boy in the world should know about.

Elmer told you how to take it off. But, most important now, he tells you *how to keep it off!*

SHE CAN'T TAKE YOU IN HER ARMS, IF SHE CAN'T GET HER ARMS AROUND YOU!—*Poor Elmer's Almanac.*

1

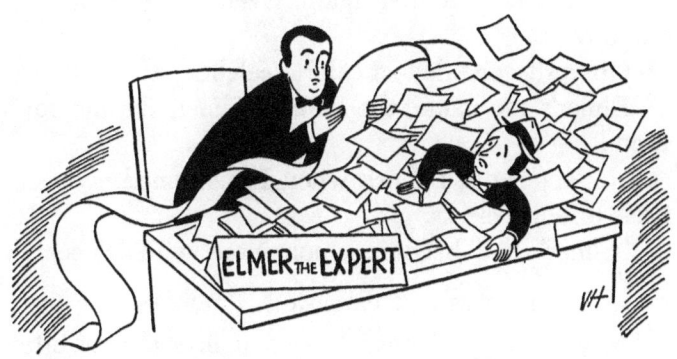

Elmer the Calorie Hero

Yippee! The world was mine!

I was a success.

Not a *huge* one, but a *thin* one.

I had written *The Fat Boy's Book,* and it broke all records!

As a serial 400 newspapers ran it, and Gallup took a poll that showed I had made 30,000,000 fatsos sit up and take notice!

Elmer the Calorie Hero

Chubby folks everywhere idolized me. I was what they hoped to be—*trim*.

Women pointed me out to their tubby hubbies and said, "Why ain't you slim, Jim, like him?"

I was a hot number again. Even my wife said so. Oh, boy!

Obscurity one day—a calorie celebrity the next.

Elmer's the name, the famous Elmer, the fat boy's friend!

No longer did I blush when I mentioned my monicker to hotel clerks.

"Elmer" had become synonymous with "Success"!

PARTIES . . . PARTIES . . . PARTIES

I never realized until I tried it myself how often people entertain a celebrity and help to fatten him up for the kill.

Nor did I realize how many "low calorie" dishes and drinks there are in the world until I was invited out to a party "In Honor of Elmer, ex-Blimp Hips!"

People noticed me on the street.

"He's the feller who wrote a best seller on how to slice off suet!"

Girls did double-takes. "There's Elmer!" they'd whisper.

I didn't have a "swoon line" of bobby-soxers, but I sure had a spoon line, not to mention knife and fork.

I hired me a secretary. Hadda keep my dates

Elmer the Calorie Hero

straight. Mustn't be at Mrs. Moe's "Trim-the-Tummy Tea" when I was due at Joe's "Juniper Juice Jag."

Yep!

All the world loves a success!

I had the public eating out of my hand—and expecting me to return the compliment about four times a day!

ELMER WOWS 'EM

But I didn't worry. It was great fun sipping the wine of success, not to mention the meat, potatoes, and desserts.

"Eggs Escoffier," beamed a host—"Spuds supreme," bragged a head waiter.

And before I could reach for my Calorie Counter they'd say, "You won't find it there, Elmer. My own low calorie invention."

"Make friends with everybody," my publisher warned me, "they're all potential buyers."

I did.

I had more free meals than a hobo. More free drinks than a Scot.

Everybody was my friend.

Like all fatsos in their forties I was sure I could pull myself down a pound or two anytime I wanted to.

My error in calculation was the "calculating calories."

Even though *I* forgot to count them, *they* were always sober enough to count themselves.

Elmer the Calorie Hero

LIFE IS MERRY!

So on I frolicked on my merry food binge. My carefree calorie caper.

Nibbling this, munching that, like a mouse in a cheese shop.

Laughing, singing, making merry.

My engagement book was filled to the brim.

So was I!

Couldn't be a heel, could I? Hadda be gracious—accept hospitality, didn't I?

Six months went by—but not unnoticed.

Success didn't go to my head. I watched that.

It didn't go to my bank account, either. Uncle Sam watched that.

Where'd it go?

You guess.

SUCCESS IS GRAND!

Sure sign of success is when the author's publisher tosses him a few parties.

Mine did. He invited in a few hand-picked reviewers. A couple of drinking columnists, a magazine staffer or two, and a lot of less fortunate authors.

They used to seek my advice on sales matters. (Remember, I'm supposed to be a sales consultant.)

Now they asked:

"What's your neck size?"

Elmer the Calorie Hero

"Your fanny?"
"How big was your pot?"
"No kiddin, Elmer! Did you really lose 40 lbs. in 80 days?"
A sad-faced author sidled up, "How'd ya ever think of such a book, anyway? Imagine! Calling fat boys fat and selling 'em a book!"
The orchestra played "The Fat Boy Bounce," * a new song I helped write.
The publisher glowed as he passed out Bering Cigars, faithfully labeled "The Fat Boy Cigar"!
I was king in his stable of authors. King—but for how long?
The hindwriting was beginning to show!

I'M A WALKING DIET BOOK

The speeches I'm invited to! Free, to be sure . . . but they are supposed to sell your book.
All I know is that back in the old B. C. days—that is, *Before Calories*—when I came to a banquet they listened to what I had to say.
Now they came to watch me eat!
In the old days they used to sit down to dinner and read the Lord's Prayer before they ate.
Now they read Elmer's Calorie Card!
No one ever dares, these days, to touch a spud or a banquet dessert (ice cream and cookie, or apple pie

* Mills Music Publishers.

Elmer the Calorie Hero

and cheese) without first waiting for the "King of Kalories" to do so first.

I loved it!

The food loved me—all too well!

Believe me it was a thrill being a calorie hero.

It can all happen so suddenly. One day you feel like the dickens, next day you feel like Dickens!

Actually I began to think I had started a new era for humanity.

The Fat Boy Reformation!

My upped status had its effect on bartenders. They'd give me free ones. "On the house," they'd say.

Then, ten minutes later, they'd sell a dozen when they whispered, "Elmer drinks 'em!"

I got news for you. Calories don't drown! They can swim!

THE CODE OF BARROOMS

What happens to a reforming fat boy at bars is a capsule course in psychology . . . and downfall.

You stop in just for a short one, and as it is going down up comes a friend. You ask him to join you.

He does. He then offers you a treat at about the time a third comes up, who must join in.

Then the third "friend" insists you have one with him. You do, and then you start things all over by buying them all a return drink. That's the code, you know!

Elmer the Calorie Hero

What started out to be a friendly appetizer on the way home turns into an evening of Nero-worship!
Friends! *Bah!*
Home drinking is the same. You stop in for "just one." Then must have another since no one is supposed to fly on one wing.
Then another for The Road.
By then, you say "What the heck," and Bacchus hangs up the flag in your honor!
The Code and The Road are hard on fat boys!

TIME PASSES NOT UNNOTICED

On I frolicked on my carefree calorie spree. Occasionally I reached for a celery instead of a calorie, but less and less as the days went on.
Occasionally I came up with some new diet information, such as, "A potato isn't any more fattening than an apple—it's the company it keeps."
That would start off a potato boom.
Then I'd crack out with, "Watermelon is often 5 times more fattening than cantaloupe!"
I'd get letters from the Watermelon Protective Association, but the Cantaloupe Gulpers Society wanted to put me in stone.
I'd quip up with such fat-boy eye-openers as, "Ya know, soft butter spreads faster than hard—and leaves you with less calories!"

Elmer the Calorie Hero

Even the butter boys liked that one!
I began to wonder how I'd really look sitting on a stone horse in the park, for posterity to ogle and envy! I was soon to learn!

IF IT TASTES GOOD, IT'S FATTENING—*Poor Elmer's Almanac.*

2

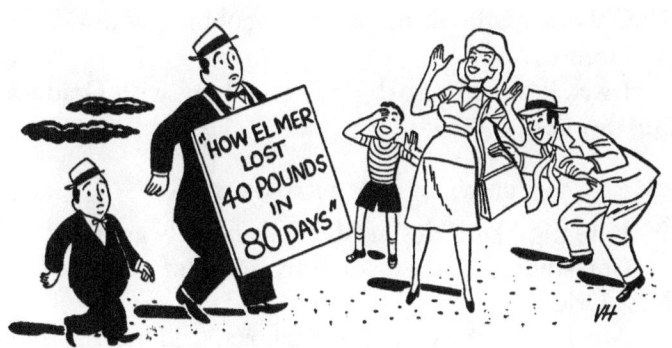

A Great Man's Critics

It was my wife who first noticed what was happening.

"Has your new suit shrunk?" she asked me one day.

"If it has," I told her, "I've wasted thirty bucks."

"Well, then," she asked, "have you stepped on the scales lately?"

"They're broke," I said.

She gave me that look a referee does when Gorgeous

A Great Man's Critics

George does something he shouldn't do, such as sticking a finger in his opponent's eye.

But considering our numbers, we Elmers do all right for ourselves.

Take Elmer, the illustrious bull. Elsie's husband.

Only he made his mark by hobnobbing with Grade-A Guernsey.

I was losing my mark by hobnobbing with Grade-A Headwaiters.

DINED BY THE BEST OF THEM

I ate pigs' knuckles at Maeder's in Milwaukee.

Got stuffed in the taxidermy room of Antoine's in New Orleans.

Ate half a steer at Toots Shor's, and hayracks of Roquefort salads at Schimmel's in Galesburg.

Lobster Southern came out of my ears at Locke-Ober's in Boston, and I drank gallons of rum concoctions at Don, the Beachcomber's.

Andy Brockles', of Dallas, where sizzling steaks originated, sent them to my house by the dozen, so instrumental was I in promoting his sales.

He'd advertise:

" 'Not a calorie in a sizzle load,' says Elmer."

I went to Keen's Chop House for their mammoth chops, and to Luchow's for their strudel.

Duncan Hines got worried!

I was becoming more of a food expert than even he.

A Great Man's Critics

ELMER'S "END" IN SIGHT

As my food piled up—so did my calories. My intake began once more to exceed my output. My metabolism began to tire out trying to burn my candles at both ends.

I began to relax—*the falling fat boy's danger signal.*

I had done a magnificent job at dieting, only to relax and brag too much, and start gaining it back.

Only an ounce a day, to be sure—but an ounce a day totals up to 23 lbs. per year!

I was six months gone.

My "end" was in sight!

And what a horrible sight it was, especially on those 12-inch seats at cocktail or milk bars.

MY FRIENDS GET AWFULLY COY

As a rapidly growing fallen fat boy, my friends began to take notice.

I began to realize I again had a weight problem when I heard a catty caddy crack with, "When he puts the ball where he can hit it, he can't see it—and when he puts it where he can see it he can't hit it."

Especially my former fat ones—ever on the alert for my downfall.

Why does all the world welcome a downfall? In fact, does everything possible to bring it about?

"What'd I tell you?" they'd chirp, "Ol' Elmer's reverting to type. *Once* a fat boy *always* a fat boy."

A Great Man's Critics

I began to be careful not to let plates gather in front of me, so it wouldn't look like I was over-eating.

I bought my collars one size larger to give the illusion of still losing weight, and I ordered belts three sizes too large just to fool my jeering fat friends gathered like buzzards around my food.

I tried to make my food disappear inconspicuously. It did. Only it didn't *stay* inconspicuous.

I often stayed awake nights wondering, "What price glory? Is it worth it?"

My wife figured it was!

MY PUBLISHER STARTS WORRYING

As my weight started up, sales of my book started down.

Gossip runs rampant. I get a letter from my publisher:

> Dear Elmer:
>
> Rumors are running around as fast as you are rounding around, that you are showing too many chins again. Say it isn't so.
>
> A book store in Kansas complains you showed up at an autograph party looking more the "before" than the "after" Elmer.
>
> Our mid-western salesman reports you waddle from banquet to banquet looking like an author who never read his book.

A *Great Man's Critics*

> A customer returns your book saying, "The man wot writ the ad shoulda writ the book. I just saw Elmer." You are the ideal of thousands of Fat Boys, Chubby Gals, and Tubby Teenagers. Don't let 'em down. Say this all isn't true.
>
> Ouch—my ulcers
> Charlie
>
> P. S.—My wife's fat girl-friend wants to know how many calories in a tomato aspic?

At first I snarled. I started to reply, dirty-like, that it was all a villainous slander cooked up by my fat friends who never took Elmer's Famous Tummy Trim, and were jealous.

Then I figured I better not. Besides, the chair I slumped into at that moment felt pretty soft.

I guess the reason Kid Kalorie was catching up again with me was I was a "poor loser."

I fell into a snooze, dreaming about a new dish I had heard about that very afternoon from the manager of the Algonquin.

I THINK UP FAT-BOY EXCUSES

My old doc, the one who got me started on my path to glory, got me started again on fat-boy excuses.

He's the guy who said, when I told him fat ran in my family, "Sure, 'cause your whole family runs to the kitchen too much!"

A Great Man's Critics

When I told him I figured it was glandular, he said there was only one gland in my body that was out of whack—my salivary gland.

I told him I ate like a bird—to which he snapped, "*Yeah—a buzzard!*"

"Furthermore," he snapped again, "it's a scientific fact that birds eat ⅓ their own weight in bird seed every day!"

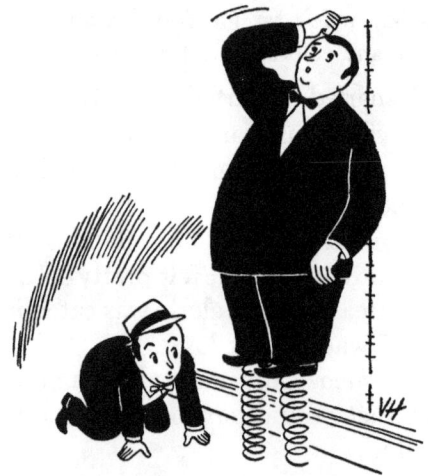

So, as a past master of fat-boy alibis, I began to think up some new ones.

When my scales showed a few extra pounds, I credited it to my "big bones." You know, insurance figures allow 10% extra weight if you're so-called big-boned.

A Great Man's Critics

All fat boys seem to be "big-boned." It's good business on their part.

I started to measure my height with my shoes on. That one inch of heel sure compensates you when you are on the downgrade—that is, *mentally*.

As winter came on, I figured it was okay to add a few pounds to get me through the winter. A neat, fallen fat-boy idea!

Don't the bears do it? I'm as smart as they, aren't I?

THE FAT BOY'S FOLLY

I could think of more excuses for getting fat again than a chef can think up low calorie dishes to ride the Fat Boy Fad.

"I guess I'm getting older," I told my doc. "Middle-age spread," I quipped, weakly.

"You should weigh at 70 the same as you weigh at 25," he snapped. "That middle-age spread idea has been exploded."

Come to think of it, you never do see a fat man aged 65—well, just a few anyway.

As a past master at calorie guzzling (I wrote the famous *Fat Boy's Book*, didn't I?), I have learned every fat-boy trick.

We fatsos can spot loopholes in insurance weight charts as quick as we can a chocolate eclair.

"Too many banquets—my business, you know," I'd

A Great Man's Critics

tell an eagle-eyed fat friend who noticed the start of another bay window on me.

Then he'd quip further, "Read your book lately, Elmer, about that famous Three-Day Calorie Counting idea!"

I got so mad at him I went into a soda fountain, and down at the end, out of sight, I drained 1,000 calories.

I'd start dieting tomorrow!

Why is it tomorrow never seems to come?

ELMER'S SWAN SONG

More and more I tried to maintain my reputation as a diet expert, especially as my speaking engagements and free meals began to peter out.

"Him—the famous fat boy!" I could hear an audience whisper, as I stood up to talk, withholding a burp.

My diet info was as good as ever. Only I had stopped practicing it as I'd crack out with such new and revealing info as:

> Just because I don't feed my dog table scraps, he has his own hair and teeth, wears no girdle, has no arch supports, has 20-20 vision—and is happy he doesn't lead "a fat boy's life."
>
> Eating at bed time puts on no more weight than eating any other time of the day—it isn't when you eat but *how* much and *how* often!
>
> Hot breads make you no fatter than cold ones. (Boy, this was exploding an old fashioned diet idea!)

A Great Man's Critics

Brick ice cream is half as fattening as hand-packed, since the air is really forced out of hand-packed.

Brother, here was *real* caloric information! Showing you how to eat—yet not gain weight. The only trouble was the bay-window set just snickered when I gave them this scientific information. My shape branded me as a phony!

IT HAPPENS TO ALL OF US

My fat boy information was still good—only I wasn't.

I had dieted, bragged, but relaxed too much and too often.

I was a backslider.

A fellow who loses 10, 15, 20 pounds, has a few months of high praise from the wife or secretary, then lets success defeat him.

For a while I tried to be philosophical. That's life, I said to myself.

Wherever you go, whatever you do, you'll find scoffers.

Try to be a bit different, I said to myself, and there's a critic aiming at you. Stick your neck out and you'll find an axe.

Only people who do things make mistakes.

Then I began feeling sorry for myself. I had started at a neat 186, and now the day had passed when I again hit 210, and was still going strong.

A Great Man's Critics

I was a fallen fat boy!

I caught myself with peanuts in my pocket, right next to my burp pills.

My wife gave up.

THE FINAL BLOW OF ALL

The night my wife gave up she served both cake and pie, neither of which is too bad for a fat boy occasionally, but not at the same sitting.

"The thing that makes me feel bad," she said, "is that there's a war coming, or on, or ending, or something—and here I am hoarding fat!"

Then a strange occurrence happened.

I was sneaking out of a new soda bar in Seattle when I ran into an old friend. We had a lot in common—15 pounds too much in common.

"I needed something to keep up my strength," I alibied, and with tolerance he nodded.

"Never mind, Elmer, old boy," he told me. "You're not the only one. There are 30,000,000 perennial fatsos, any one of whom can take it off. But we always let it come back on!"

Do we?

We do?

And I wondered why?

> BLIMPS ARE MADE AT BLOWOUTS—*Poor Elmer's Almanac.*

3

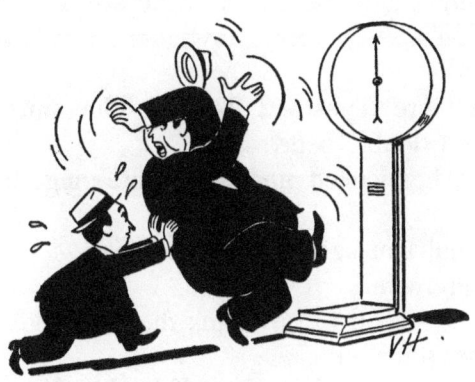

The Hindwriting on Elmer's Breadbasket

My crown was toppling under an assault of calories.

Instead of "Your Majesty" the fat boys were beginning to call me "Your Lardship."

Again I was fast becoming a hippo of the hash house, a café colossus.

A fallen fat boy, one who dieted, bragged, but relaxed too much and began to gain it back.

All because I tried to be a great guy—a good sport.

The Hindwriting on Elmer's Breadbasket

My weight went up, my popularity went down. I sagged along with my bay window.

I used to be athletic—now I'm apathetic.

I couldn't look the scales in the eye. In fact, it got so I couldn't see the scales any more around the breadbasket.

Once more I yearned for dark blue suits, fat-boy chairs, and double beds.

My arches looked up at the gathering storm. My downfall.

"Oh, no! Not again!" they screamed.

And my wife?

Well, she tried to buy back the twin beds she had sold to her sorority!

"Have you looked at yourself lately—sidewise?" she sneered.

AN EZIO PINZA HAIRCUT

Fat-boy psychology is darned interesting.

Take the haircut, for example. Feeling like a fallen hero, I visited my barber.

I pulled myself up as erect as I could, as I walked in wondering maybe I should buy some Adlers after all. That extra inch would allow me another few pounds of weight.

I kept telling myself that I wasn't too heavy—just not tall enough.

My barber's hand twitched nervously while he lis-

The Hindwriting on Elmer's Breadbasket

tened to my sad tale. I had him down 10 pounds, and now he was up 12.

So he wasn't too kindly toward me these days, but still had to earn an honest buck.

"Got you," he said at length, after I tried to explain the illusion I tried to get him to create. "What you want is a little higher on the sides, less on the top—gives you that thin-boy look!"

"Not a brush haircut," I warned, "like them TV announcers."

When I got home that night, sporting my short haircut, the wife takes a double look at me and screams in mirth:

"Look," she howls to Martha the cook, "Old Lard Face is making like Ezio Pinza!"

Not long after that I reverted back to cream and sugar in my coffee!

ELMER'S A FAT-BOY FRAUD

For a while I had figured I was a Fat-Boy Freud! Now I began to realize I was just a Fraud!

You don't have to go to college to know more than your doctor. All you need is to be sick.

Maybe you don't know about as many different kinds of ailments. You don't have to. All you care about is what ails *you*.

That was the way with me. When I became interested in reducing, I went after facts. I read books. I

The Hindwriting on Elmer's Breadbasket

talked to dietitians. I listened to doctors. And soon I could talk like an expert.

I *was* an expert.

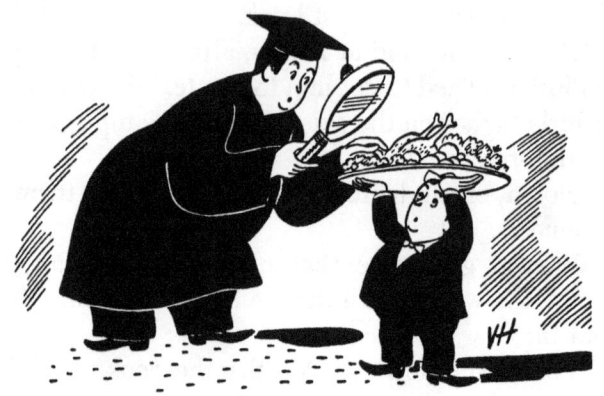

I could reel off facts to make your head spin, like these:

> Green olives are half as fattening as black ones.
>
> Stale bread crumbles on the table, so less calories get into you than when you eat fresh bread.
>
> The lighter the beer—the less calories. In fact, some beers today are often less per ounce than many pops.
>
> Tomatoes are more slenderizing than turnips, even though a Broadway play glamorized the turnip.

The Hindwriting on Elmer's Breadbasket

I HAD ALL THE RIGHT ANSWERS

That's what made me wonder why I was expanding again.

Must you?

Can't you lose weight—yet not gain it back? With some fatsos gaining twice back as if the rebound sent them even more skyward?

Nothing I can do about currency inflation, but if I could check fat boy inflation, I might again become The Fat Boy's Hero.

So I figured out a couple of posers for me, Elmer the Expert.

Is it true that Fat Boys, their chubby mates, and tubby teenagers, after taking it off, usually gain it all back?

And if so, why?

The answer to this great question lies deeper than diet.

A GREAT MAN THINKS ON

Your doc can tell you to take it off, I can tell you how to take it off,

A psychiatrist, maybe?

"You have given me food for thought," one psychiatrist said when I suggested he open a fallen fat boy's department.

He described his methods.

The Hindwriting on Elmer's Breadbasket

It seems you lie on a couch and you tell him all that is on your mind. He gets clues from your past that might tell why you are fat.

You're bound to spill something that gives you away.

But what could that doc make out of my words that would be a mystery?

All I'd perhaps think would be, say, "chocolate eclair," "guinea hen under glass," "veal cutlets," "lobster Newburg."

MORE FOOD FOR THOUGHT

It's an intellectual method, and does a lot of good. But I was curious about more than just myself.

If my regaining lost fat was the exception to the rule, I'd know what to do about it.

But if mine was a common experience, that of dieting and gaining it all back, I wanted to find out why it happens to all of us.

How come Gallup could dig up so easily 30,000,000 fatsos even in these days of eggs at a buck and butter nearly as high?

But I was tempted, before going further into research, to take up that couch expert's suggestion, and talk.

But I better not have my wife around.

I overheard the wife tell a neighbor my trouble was I was eating "like a growing boy, only he is growing frontwards and backwards."

The Hindwriting on Elmer's Breadbasket

On second thought, maybe I'd better not be around either.

I was afraid of that couch.

In my present bloated condition, it looked too good!

THE STRAW THAT BREAKS FATSO'S BACK

I had a lot of fun thinking this way, but a bowl of stew that passed my nose at the athletic club stopped these thoughts.

Then one of the club's directors spotted me eating behind a palm plant, and with all seriousness asked would I like to be the kids' Santa Claus this year.

"We need a famous man—a big one," he said seriously.

Two days later I was down at the far end of a soda fountain, hidden, I thought, behind a 12-inch banana split, when I was spied by another sneaking fatso.

"Ah, ah!" he smirked, "mustn't touchy!"

I winced like a reformed pickpocket who finds a purse on the street about the time a cop happens by and somebody shouts, "I've been robbed!"

My friend snorted and yanked one of my calorie cards from his pocket.

"Fake," he sneered, as he tore it up, and joined me in a 12-inch banana split.

Only he had Brazil nuts on top of his.

The Hindwriting on Elmer's Breadbasket

SO ELMER FACES FACTS

As I trudged off down the street I had to face the facts.

The Fat Boy was back again.

In person.

That couch idea began to sound good after all—especially to my arches.

Yes, sir, I was plenty worried by now about my mental attitude.

Was I trying to pen up a Fatso's mind in a Slim Jim's body?

Was it a case that for a while my body got slim but my spirits stayed roly-poly?

Why was I gaining it all back?

NO EXERCISE FOR ELMER

Exercises have never bothered me. I can watch people take calisthenics for hours.

I just can't watch 'em take calories for one minute.

I remembered my own advice, before I got the exercise urge, that "Exercise makes muscles loose, but in itself will not reduce."

Of course, a little physical effort does everybody good. Trouble was, I got mine walking from my car into famous restaurants.

It was my swan song—and I planned to make the most of it, before I started back to dieting—tomorrow.

The Hindwriting on Elmer's Breadbasket

So for a month more I ate kidney stew in wine at the Royal York in Toronto, snails served in stew at Hotel Emporio in Mexico City, and octopus tails in sherry at La Louisian in Monterey.

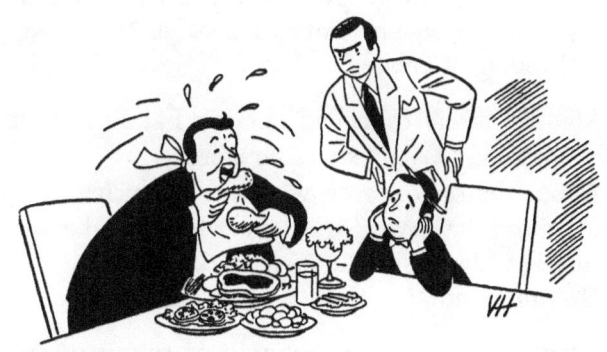

Jumbo salads at Hotel Roosevelt in Hollywood, and in every city where there is a Statler I made away with their famous rum-bottom pie.

And there are a lot of cities with Statler Hotels, too.

Soon, when I heard anybody say, "Bottoms up!" I thought they were getting personal!

FAT BOYS CAN'T FOOL ANYBODY

By now it was six months since my book had become a meteoric success.

Six fun-filled months.

The Hindwriting on Elmer's Breadbasket

I get my second letter from my publisher. He had given up.

Dear Elmer:

Maybe we'd better forget about further diet books. The fad seems to have fizzled out. How about starting a new rage by writing a book on "The Care and Feeding of Public Speakers"?

Manufacturers cancelled out my Fat Boy testimonials. Hopalong Calories was no more.

About the only person who was really happy with Elmer these days was Sig Klein, who runs the world-famous Fat Man's Shop in New York City.

He ran an ad:

ELMER'S BACK AGAIN. BUSINESS IS SPREADING

PASS UP THE FIRST ROLL—YOU'LL ALWAYS GET A SECOND—
Poor Elmer's Almanac.

4

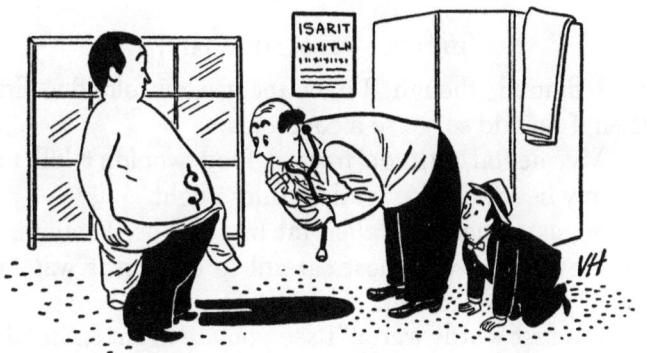

Elmer Returns to His Doc

Yes, sir, I was plenty worried by now about my mental attitude.

Was I the singer who always wanted to dance, the dancer who always yearned to sing?

Why is it the fiddler wants to play the drums, and the business man wants to be the clown at the circus?

What is this peculiar twist in us fat boys that makes us look into mirrors and long to see ourselves dressed like Adolph Menjou?

I began to feel persecuted.

Elmer Returns to His Doc

Everybody was watching me—just hoping I'd make one false move.

That's it. I was persecuted!

Maybe I'd better see that psychiatrist.

"HI, DOC——IT'S ME AGAIN!"

I figured, though, I'd better see my old doc first, then if he said so, go to a couch man.

My mental attitude toward food wouldn't kill me, but my heart, liver, or gall bladder might.

So, as casual as a fallen fat boy can be, I sauntered into my doc. I was most careful to explain it was just for a "yearly check up."

His first words were: "I see you are again eating like a king—four kings." While my doc is a learned cuss, he isn't above sarcasm.

"So you're the bird who wrote a book on how to fight fat with knowledge," he said. "My, my! You sure piled on more *muscles!*"

I hefted up my excess baggage in order to assert myself, but he banged my knee with a hammer.

"Well, you ain't crazy—*yet!*" he said, as my leg flew against my bay window. "Maybe just silly—but not entirely nuts."

My blood-shot eyes were blazing, but at least he settled that psychiatrist question.

I told the doc it wasn't that I weighed too much, but that I was not tall enough.

Elmer Returns to His Doc

"You ought to know," he kept on, "being overweight is like carrying your own death warrant around."

"More suicides are fat!"

"Thought you'd put us docs outa business, didn't you," he sneered—"writing a book on how to lose weight and have fun?"

I protested, "Didn't I keep telling people to see their doc?"

"Who's gonna believe a big lard-can like you?" he countered. "Please do me a real favor and don't tell people I'm your doc. I'd lose their trade!"

Then he grabbed my own book off the shelf.

HE READS ME THE DIET ACT

"Listen, you Blimp Boy, there isn't anything wrong with you that less food won't cure!"

Then he proceeds to tell me—right from my own book, mind you—that the reason fat boys diet and regain weight is because they start eating too much again.

"But why?" I ask, "why do they lose weight, enjoy the pleasures, then give up and gain it back?"

"For several reasons," he goes on, and really wises me up.

His first big reason was that too many fat folks diet too fast. They go on a diet binge, knock off 10 pounds, but are so darned hungry that when the binge is over they eat like two horses, instead of one.

If they'd lose weight slower, they'd be less hungry

Elmer Returns to His Doc

when the diet stage is over with, and have less urge to rush for the pantry shelf yelling, "The diet's over! the diet's *over!*"

I GET SOME SENSIBLE ADVICE

"It says here in your book, fat boy," goes on the doc, "that a spoonful of salt keeps a pint of water in the body. How's your salt content, lately?"

He and I both know it's about the same as the Pacific Ocean.

I asked the doc why *he* doesn't write a book on losing weight, in language fat boys, their chubby mates, and tubby teenagers would understand.

I think I have him there. But he comes back with, "If I did—*I'd practice it!*"

Then he storms on:

"You gained weight because you didn't allow your system to get used to its new weight. You did a good job at dieting, but didn't keep it up long enough. Being a calorie hero went to your head! Well—other places, too!"

He had something there. When your system remembers too well the fat foods, it is hard to keep your mind off them.

Your whole body has an urge for food. You are fighting years of eating, of overfeeding the body. And it craves food like an alcoholic craves whiskey!

Elmer Returns to His Doc

YOU HAVE OTHER THINGS ON YOUR MIND

Yes, sir, I learned a lot about why fat people have their downfalls.

Not only does the body crave the fat nourishment it has been accustomed to, but so does your mind.

But memory is short. After you hold your present weight for three months (six are better), then your mind is off food, and on other things.

Once you can get up and at 'em again, you are apt to be more interested in a brace of blonde legs than chicken wings!

This keeps you on the go.

Naturally you burn up more food moving around this way as a thin boy, back in the mood, than as a fatso filled with vittles and slumped in the old man's club.

YOU FORM NEW EATING HABITS

What is more, if you don't go on a quickie diet, but a long-term, sensible one, you have a chance to learn new habits in eating.

Like the crook sent up for 30 days. He hasn't learned new habits. Keep him up for 3 months, and maybe he has learned the habit of honesty.

You were not born to like chocolate eclairs. You cultivated this habit. Maybe by watching your fat gross mudder.

Chinese weren't born to like Chow Mein—nor were

Elmer Returns to His Doc

you born to like steaks. You each cultivated that "habit" from your family, and national custom.

So when you take on a long-term diet, like a long-term wife, you learn new habits.

You learn to like coffee black. You really taste it. You learn to like thinner soups, and are content with half a loaf instead of a whole loaf.

You become a gourmet instead of a gourmand!

THE DOC'S PARTING SHOT

Indeed, that doc sure knew his groceries! Trouble was I knew too many groceries!

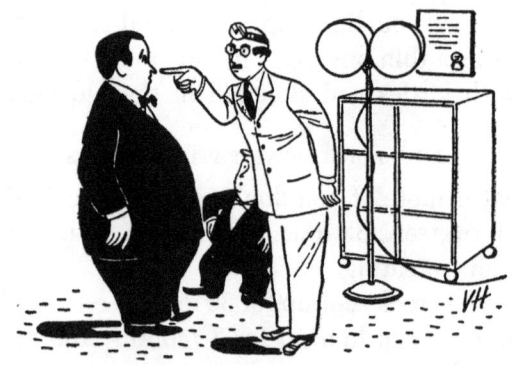

As a parting shot he said, "Take that schnozzle of yours. It's a beautiful but horrible example of high-blood-pressure red! I see you didn't remember that alcohol is liquid calories."

Elmer Returns to His Doc

I wanted to say something about The Code and The Road, but he cut me short. Being fat again, my reflexes had slowed up. I was no mental equal to this thin-size sawbones.

"Naturally," he said, "an orange juice has more calories than a Scotch and soda, as you so nicely brought out in your book, but even the newest member of the A. A. can figure that five Scotches have more calories than one morning orange juice."

That guy was so horribly right! Like my wife!

THE CHINESE PUZZLE

The longer I stayed with old Sawbones, the more I respected the fellow.

He sure was a bag of bones—but he wasn't any fathead.

He knew his calories, but most of all he knew his fatsos.

I guess he had seen lard faces like me come and go, and come back!

He didn't fill me up with the old stuff about the exercise that counts most is pushing yourself from the table.

Nor did he give me the old stuff about shaking the head sidewise will do more to keep off weight than raising weights.

His problem, on hand, was a typical fatso who won

Elmer Returns to His Doc

his laurels by slicing off a 40 pound sack of suet—but then what to do to keep it off?

I had won my Purple Heart by doing something noble beyond the call of the dinner bell, but had slumped.

I was a puzzle. Or was I?

Anyhow, there are 30,000,000 of us!

What would you give to lose your second suitcase a second time?

LEARNING TO KEEP IT OFF

I had gone merrily down the primrose path to the Land of Oz.

And 16 ozs. make a pound, you know.

Now it was time to hit the road back.

Only that morning the wife had cracked out with, "On the way home, Fat Boy, drop in and see if they sell such things as rubber thread."

When I fell for the gag and asked what was the idea of rubber thread, she sneered, "For the buttons in your shirt-collar—I've moved them to the very edge!"

Which is why this doc, with his fat-boy advice on how to keep it off once it is off, interested me.

Come to think of it, if you don't eat a certain food for a long time, you do lose the taste for it. At least, it becomes lost in your memory.

But that first diet-week, boy, how I dreamed all day long about waffles and maple syrup, smothered in bacon!

Elmer Returns to His Doc

As time went on, the dream melted away, much like the vision of that beautiful redhead when you were twenty.

So I guess old doc is right, and here are three rules for keeping it off:

RULE 1 for keeping it off is:

Don't Take It Off Too Fast

The slower it goes off—the slower it comes back on. It took you 10 years maybe to pack it on—so don't expect it to roll off in 10 days.

RULE 2. *Keep It Off Six Months*

By this time, unless you are a born glutton, you will lose some of the urge for icings, sugar in the coffee, and a dozen doughnuts to one cup of black coffee.

RULE 3. *Develop New Eating Habits*

That's it. Learn to like *new* foods—those with fewer calories in them.

Do you know how to tell a calorie-packed food? If you like it—*it's bound to be fattening.*

That's the test any fatso puts to his food.

NEW HOPE FOR ELMER

Hope begins to come back to me.

Perhaps I can again become the Savior of Fatsos!

Elmer Returns to His Doc

A new Pied Piper of Lard Faces!

A Joan of Arc for fatsos with the desire but not the will.

A Carrie Nation agin' Carrying Calories!

Gosh, maybe that stone statue in the park ain't a dream after all.

I raise myself up from the doc's comfortable chair ... with a little help from him.

"Better tie your shoelaces, Fat Boy," he says, as we part, "and pull your collar back into place."

He helps me on with my coat. I guess he saw that hope had risen in my bourbon-tinted eyes.

A FAT BOY IN YOUR FUTURE

I wobble down the street, thinking.

I was thinking so hard I passed three bakery windows without realizing it.

A skinny friend of mine quipped, "Matter, Elmer, got a calorie jag on? You passed up a window of cheese cake."

"Okay, smart boy," I yelped back on him, "remember there's a fat boy in your future!"

His face fell. I guess he figured he never wanted ever to look like me.

But I'd show them. I had a vision that day. I'd again become the Savior of Fatsos. Might even start a Fallen Fat Boys' Shrine!

The Fat Boys' friend—a haven of fallen fat boys.

Elmer Returns to His Doc

Their downfall would become my hobby in life. I'd find out why people can't lose weight, and not gain it back.

I'd use the Salvation Army slogan, "A man may be down, but he's never out!"

That night Martha stirred up a cocktail full of potent and brought in a giant-size tray of hors d'oeuvres.

I shook my head no—dramatically.

"What is you, man or *mouse?*" she asked, disgustedly.

Abashed, I took a big hunk of cheese!

A GUEST AND A CALORIE ANNOY ON THE THIRD DAY—*Poor Elmer's Almanac.*

5

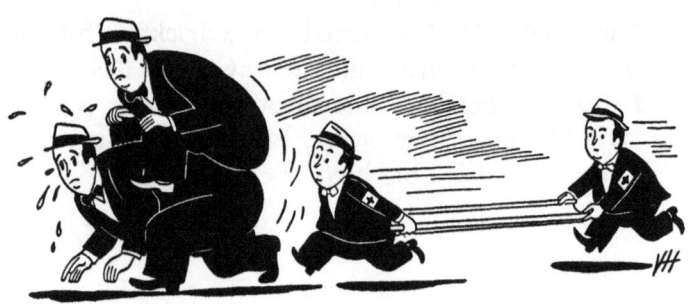

Elmer Rises Out of the Ashes

I felt like that bird that rose out of the ashes. Was it a pelican or eagle or something?

Anyhow, I had found a goal in life: to save fatsos from an early grave!

I had told them how to take it off—now I must find rules and methods and systems to show them how to keep it off.

"I can lose 10 lbs. any day I want," is the favorite beef of the fatso. "Only when I stop dieting I gain it all back—and more!"

Elmer Rises Out of the Ashes

I had found the reason why from my doc.

Now I must delve further into the psychology of why fat folks are fat!

I'd devote my life to it!

My very own fat!

I LOOK FOR FERDY FLUBB

I needed help in my one-man war against bulges.

Birds of a feather flock together, so I went to look up an old pal of mine, Fatso Ferdy.

I knew Ferdy had read my book and had removed a mezzanine he'd been toting around for years.

We had lots of fun for a month or two showing our "bragging belts" to our friends, and our horse-collared shirts.

Whenever somebody said, "I paid $20,000 to install my bay window—how much *you* willing to give me to lose it?" Ferdy and I had our answers.

We told the guy did he know that for every one per cent overweight he was he'd die one per cent sooner?

That if he was 25 per cent overweight at 45 he'd die 25 per cent sooner?

That 80 per cent of all diabetics were once fat boys —and that docs now find that a majority of "heart troubles" are due to the heart's pushing and shoving all day long in layers of fat?

And that for every one inch his tummy stood out in front of his chest, he'd die one year sooner?

Elmer Rises Out of the Ashes

That these were facts from the American Medical Association boys, and if he didn't believe it, the first insurance man he'd meet would soon convince him!

After all, insurance sellers don't place book on losing facts! Just losing fat!

I FIND FERDY

So I wanted to find Ferdy. Maybe he could help me pull myself back into shape and become a Fat Boy Apostle for my newest crusade against Death by Lard!

I went to his hotel.

The lobby was empty except for one tremendous fatso parked in an easy chair over by the pot plants. That's near the dining room, which still wasn't due to open for an hour.

I started toward the house phones to call Ferdy, when the hunk of fatso stirred, like a water buffalo wallowing to its feed in an African thicket.

"Hey, fat boy," wheezed the lard face. "Watsa matter, getting too famous to speak to an old friend!"

My gosh! It was Ferdy!

WHAT MADE FERDY FAT?

Here was where to start. With an old fat friend—a two-time loser.

So I started in to analyze Ferdy. I fed him well that night to soften him up for my kill, like you give drinks to a drunkard you want to rob.

Elmer Rises Out of the Ashes

Ferdy Flubb told me he still felt fit as a fiddle. He must have meant a bass fiddle.

Analyzing a true, dyed-in-the-wool fatso is interesting.

Once they admit they are fat, then they start bragging on it, like a fellow stuck with a lemon car.

Did you know a fat boy eats his own weight in food every six weeks?

Imagine Ferdy Flubb eating 280 pounds of food every month and a half!

Fat boys try to walk faster, to leap up steps, to put on a great show of not being heavy-hoofed.

They are inclined to wear overly-tight suits, *fat boy falsies*, to give the illusion of being less weighty.

They love to be thought jolly. They sneak a burp pill into them, and before it has time to resound, out pops a new story to hide the bang.

They are all front-parlor medical experts. They know all the latest in burp pills.

They make continual fun of skinny boys, like the poor man does of the rich man.

They have inferiority complexes.

When a fat friend goes on a diet, they say he looks weak, sick, horrible.

They tell his friends he had to: ". . . disease" . . . "family troubles" . . . "financial worries."

Fat boys are an interesting study, like the Wiffle Birds at zoos!

Elmer Rises Out of the Ashes

SO IT WAS WITH FERDY

I had heard all the fat-boy beefs and alibis for years, but now I was studying the "why" behind the alibis.

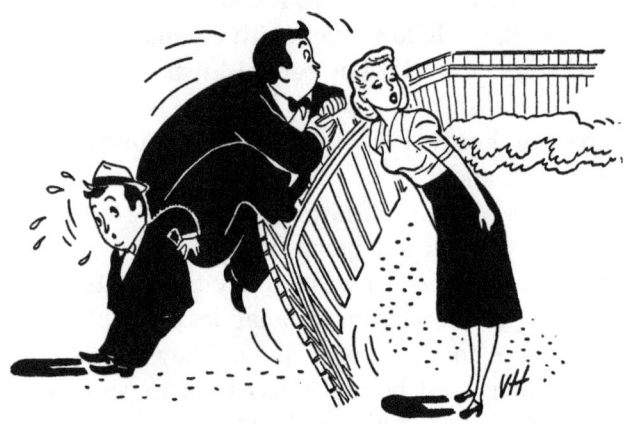

I guess the three hardest things in the world to do are: kiss a girl when she leans away from you; climb a fence that leans toward you; or stay a thin boy with fat friends kidding you.

I sure was in no shape myself to bawl out Ferdy.

I listened to Ferdy for an hour, until finally he stopped eating and went off to sleep until breakfast time.

I started back home, dejected. But I was determined to find the answers, and so started right in on some real research.

Elmer Rises Out of the Ashes

I started to analyze fatsos as they passed me by, and finally came up with these categories. There must be some 57 varieties, but here are a few I saw on the way home from Ferdy's:

Torpedo Type: He has a pot belly, his sole distinguishing claim for the fat boy award. A belly like the warhead on a submarine missile. He is fond of Morris chairs. You'll find him in Officers' Clubs between wars—and meals.

Penguin: He waddles as he walks. His legs are short like pier pilings. His body is long and has the general aspect of a pillbox on the Maginot line. He has his own battle line now. It's bulging. People scatter when he meets them on sidewalks.

Razorback: So named for his resemblance to that breed of Arkansas hog. His legs are long and slender, his back lean. But from his jowls down he is solid suet. You often find him in the stock exchange.

Diamond Jim Brady: The really big fellow. Six foot of food—and all fat. He calls it muscles. He got them, he says, playing football for Old Yale. Pockets bulging with due bills, deputy sheriff's badges, and burp pills.

Barrel Chest: A type found on upper Broadway. Usually in front of the Brill Building, Tin Pan Alley, home of the new recording, "The Fat Boy Bounce."

Steamer Trunk Derrieres: Heavy on the rear, mainly. From too much sitting. You find them in front of rou-

Elmer Rises Out of the Ashes

lette wheels in Reno. They are very noticeable in their store-bought "out-where-the-West-begins" regalia.

Kitchen Sneak: Psychiatrists have found a new type of fatso. The "kitchen sneak." He pretends to help at parties, only every time he goes to the kitchen "to help" —he does! He helps himself to a handful of calories. "Sneaks" often complain they never eat. They "sneak" instead.

ONE THING IS PLAIN

I have a good yearly crop of fat boys on which to work. That's as plain as their hind ends.

When you see seamen without a home, you make them one; you take juveniles off the streets and educate them; and even form a haven for barber shop singers.

Why not a fat boys' society? A "home" for fallen fat boys—maybe even a fat boys' farm?

A place where they can be studied, like ants. A spot, free of poison ivy, where they can be taught the evils of calories.

A place where they can fight their fat problems together. United, they can fight Kid Kalorie. Separately, they are a civic problem.

Misery loves company, so I sure ought to be able to get a fat flock together for my scientific research into why fat boys diet twice a year, yet gain it all back.

Father Elmer's own "Fat Boys' Town."

A Fat Boys' Institute of America!

Elmer Rises Out of the Ashes

FEED THEM SCIENTIFIC MEDICINES

Here I could feed them scientific "medicines." Aren't they as "sick" as alcoholics? Isn't a thirst for calories as harmful to society as for overdoses of whiskey or sleeping pills?

I'd scare them with such facts as:

> For every pound of fat you add, you add also one mile of *extra blood vessels* for the heart to pump blood through.
>
> If you are 40 lbs. overweight . . . you have 40 *extra miles* of pipes for the old heart to pump the nectar of life through!

I'd scare the suet off them.

No medicines. No exercise. Just knowledge of what happens when you are too fat.

Then real information on how to "eat away" the fat!

MORE RULES TO KEEP IT OFF

Yes, sir, I'd feed my pack of fatsos with knowledge such as:

Rule 1: Don't Make Dieting a Guessing Game. If you have to guess what is in food, you are apt to get a caloric punch in the bread basket you don't expect. Eating isn't a gamble. You can guess wrong too often—too late.

Rule 2: Fight Fat With Knowledge. You can remove the guess and gamble out of what to eat with knowledge. Know-

Elmer Rises Out of the Ashes

how. Looking at a smörgåsbord and knowing you can eat caviar (25 calories); lobster (75); halibut (150)—and not knock yourself out.

Rule 3: Form the Habit of NOT Eating. Since eating is a habit, why not form a habit of NOT eating? Simple logic? But how? Well, making the boys blonde-happy again might divert their attention, but showing them low caloried foods might work just as well until they get back on their feet.

ELMER GETS GOING IN HIGH GEAR

Maybe I'll form a Helping Hand Society, too, for those who can't come to the farm.

You know, here you sit some night facing a plate of pigs' knuckles and dumplings, with cake, pie, and cheese.

You have a phone number to call.

"Hey, Charlie," you cry over the phone, "come quick. I need help."

Charlie, a chosen-in-advance Slim Jim, then rushes over and lends a helping hand.

He eats half the food so that the fat victim-in-need isn't slugged quite so badly.

Great idea!

Better practice this myself, I think.

For I had gotten so I was eating a barrel of food again—and looking like the barrel.

I had begun to love gravy, and gravy, you know,

Elmer Rises Out of the Ashes

comes from the Greek restaurant word meaning "Grave Yard!"

I'd quit hobnobbing with Omar, the tent man.

No more would clerks send me to the Fat Man's Dept. Imagine me, Elmer, Captain in the Marine Corps, Y. M. C. A. director, *Eagle Scout*—en route to the Fat Man's Dept.!

H-m-m . . .

Wonder what a fellow does about the pigeon situation when they carve him on stone and place him in a public park . . .

IF AND WHEN YOU NO LONGER SAG,
THEN SURE AS HECK YOU'VE A RIGHT TO BRAG
—*Poor Elmer's Almanac.*

6

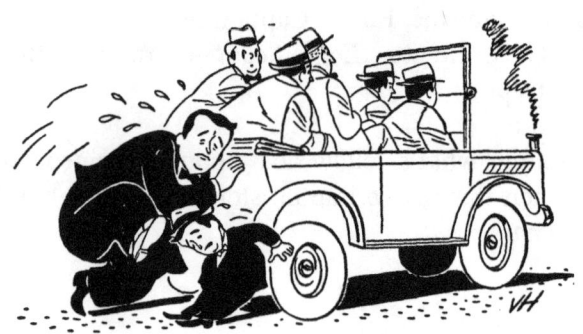

Elmer Organizes the F.B.I.
(Fat Boys' Institute)

When I returned from my visit with Ferdy, fixed in my determination to do something about fallen fatsos who need a booster to keep them going, I came smack into Martha, our 300-lb. cook.

My home is in the station wagon, saddle, and septic tank part of Dallas, Texas. The high-caloric end of town. The Hypochondriac Belt.

Elmer Organizes the F. B. I.
The maids, therefore, are all well-fed.
Martha was always one to exaggerate, but when she greeted me with, "Law, you sure look like a wayward pussy cat," I caught the point and got mad.
Shame in my own castle.
That afternoon the postman arrived with a rejection slip for a diet article.
After getting fat I was beginning to write under the name of Imogene Kerplogsky to food editors.
The postman smiled as he handed me the obvious rejection slip, remarking, "For you, Imogene!"
So then and there I organized The Fat Boys' Institute.

PURPOSE OF THE F. B. I.

Knowledge prevents many a disease. So I figured this same idea of exposing fat boys to knowledge would help them cure themselves.
The purpose of our F. B. I. would be to combat crime at the dinner table. To perpetuate fat boys by thinning them out.
I reasoned that as knowledge helped fight malaria, so knowledge of Kid Kalorie would help fallen fat boys from becoming full and complete downfalls.
Especially fatsos overly susceptible to Siamese chins.
We'd do this not with machines or exercise or harmful drugs, just a knowledge of what to eat and what to side-step.

Elmer Organizes the F. B. I.

A noble undertaking! I got a letter of endorsement from the head statistician of an insurance firm.

"We'll have more customers to sell when you finish your National Tummy Trims," they wrote, enclosing a due bill for a policy "when you've made the grade, yourself."

ONE OF OUR FAT-BOY TRICKS

The reason why fatso reverts to fat after a diet spree is because of one word—"no."

Everything he likes his wife says, "No—it'll make you fat!"

But with Elmer and his Fat Boys' Institute, it will be different.

We're gonna be "Yes men"!

I'll teach 'em what to eat—instead of what not to eat—so they will hear only "Yes—eat that" instead of "No—that's forbidden."

It will be:

"Yes—a lobster is no more fattening than a fried egg!"
"Yes—asparagus has only 5 calories—you can eat a dozen!"
"Yes—a baked spud is okay with one patty of butter!"
"Yes—you need starch to burn up meat—so eat bread!"
"Yes—butter's your friend when you don't offend."
"Yes—go on a candy binge but know what you've done!"

Elmer Organizes the F. B. I.

People taking Elmer's Booster Course for Fallen Fat Boys—those who dieted, relaxed, but gained it back—will love this "Yes Method"!

SOME EARLY RESEARCH

There are two ways to make a fallen fat boy regret and start him back on the right road. To get him off the High Calorie Wagon:

1. Take him to a musical comedy and let him ogle all the pretty girls. He will sigh and regret that they no longer yearn for him, that it is a fallacy that "everybody loves a fat man."

   Fat men are not loved. Who can love a hunk of lard, sweating in the heat, puffing from a dance, burping from a meal, sleeping after a dinner?

   He'll either be shocked into dieting by this treatment, or go down and drown his sorrows in more food!

2. Way number two is to scare old baggy pants into dieting. When he is under 35 this is hard to do. His system can throw off tons of suet troubles, and his heart can stand the gait. But after 35 he breaks down.

Just like a car after 40,000 miles. You don't run it so fast up hills, or it boils over. Load it up with a few fat boys and its arches spring. So maybe here is our best way to force fatso into taking Elmer's Calorie Cure.

I get the low-down on fat-boy troubles from my doc.

Elmer Organizes the F. B. I.

FAT-BOY OCCUPATIONAL HAZARDS

Here is the horrible list, straight from the doc's medicine cabinet, of where fatso can look for his future trouble:

1. The Heart.
2. The Gall Bladder.
3. Diabetes.
4. High Blood Pressure.
5. The Kidneys.
6. The Liver.
7. Allergies.
8. Fallen Arches.
9. Depression Psychosis.

Take the heart.

Newest discoveries indicate fat clustered around the heart is a major cause of many "heart troubles."

Maybe the old adage ought to be written this way:

"Eat, drink, and be merry too often—and tomorrow you'll die for sure."

I'm told the heart was made to last more than 100 years.

But a heart doused perpetually in pies, liverwurst, dumplings, and alcohol gives up life early for a pair of wings.

An army may travel on its stomach, as Napoleon once said, but us fat boys sure can't travel far on ours.

THE GALL BLADDER AND LIVER

Body mechanisms are amazing things. How complicated and hard-working they are!

Elmer Organizes the F. B. I.

The liver is a sort of chemical plant that manufactures bile, which is then stockpiled (in true government fashion) inside the gall bladder.

You send down a few hamburgers, and the gall bladder sends out a squirt of bile to help digest the 'burgers and remove some of the burp from the onions and pickles.

Bile is needed especially by fat boys for their fat foods, so when you overeat from the frying pan, your gall bladder gets an extra workout. It doesn't like that. It gets weary of squirting out bile.

Then your liver goes on a sympathy strike and slows up the manufacturing end of the business.

Soon the fried oysters, chicken, French-fries, and hash-browns find a bile shortage. So they move on into your innards "half-biled" (if there is such a word).

Result: The fat boy's distress signal goes out.

The burp!

So our F. B. I. quickly grabbed this jingle from *Poor Elmer's Almanac:*

>Cheer the host who serves the roast,
>But run and hide from food that's fried.

THE FAT BOY AND DIABETES

As a fat boy, I was always leery of diabetes.

It's just too much sugar where it shouldn't be.

"Diabetes is more prevalent among fat people than thin people," my doc says.

Elmer Organizes the F. B. I.

Every time I got thirsty I figured I had diabetes, because it's thirst that's supposed to be Sign No. 1. (Still, my Uncle Albert had a thirst that took 50 years to quench, and he never had diabetes.)

I learned, though, that diabetes, unlike weight, can pass from one generation to another. So ask your Aunt Suzie if she has it. That's a good clue for you to follow.

Diet, I was advised, is the best way to control diabetes. And if you do as the doc advises, you'll probably live to be 100!

HIGH BLOOD PRESSURE AND FAT BOYS

"Everybody has blood pressure," doc tells me. "The $64 question is *how much do you have?*"

Blood goes through your arteries at a certain pressure.

If the arteries harden, the pressure goes up.

Old age and wrong eating harden the tubes. We can't do anything about growing older but try to do it gracefully—and that means, for one thing, eating properly.

THE FAT BOY'S KIDNEYS

The kidneys' purpose seems to be to drain the poisons from our systems, especially poisons that accumulate as the result of over-eating and over-drinking.

They're a kind of sieve.

But, like an automatic dishwasher in the kitchen,

Elmer Organizes the F. B. I.

they won't last a lifetime if they are working all the time.

ALLERGIES AND OLD FATSO

Putting on excess weight means putting extra work on the various moving or non-moving parts of the body. (And Fatso's are mostly *non*-moving.)

It's like dumping a load of fat friends into your car. The old bus just naturally won't steer as well. The tires will wear out faster, and soon the pistons pant to an early end on some steep hill.

By over-working the body—wrapping it in layers of superfluous suet—you tire it out. You make it easy prey for "fat-boy nerves" and allergies.

Ever notice the "fat boy's twitch"?

Unconsciously, he often twists his neck or arms—or winks when there isn't even a pretty gal in sight.

His nerves are weary from a fat overload. Like an over-loaded electric wire—he blows a fuse.

Allergies love to pester fat boys. Faces swell from even such common foods as milk, wheat, or eggs.

A healthy body would toss off the allergy. But our fat bodies are just too lazy—too bogged down to fight for us.

So, in the front row of some clinic you sigh to yourself: "And fat boys are supposed to be jolly. Bah!"

Elmer Organizes the F. B. I.

FATTY'S SCREAMING ARCHES

The fat boy's favorite pose is sitting on the edge of a chair (softest in the place) trying to hoist one foot over his bay window so he can nurse his protesting arches.

It stands to reason: if you carry a 40-lb. sack of suet on your torso all day long your arches aren't going to be friendly.

Once you drop 10, 15 or 40 pounds your arches feel springy again. The fat boy's waddle and wobble disappear.

If you keep a *munch-by-munch* record on the Fat Boy's Thermometer, your waddle will soon vanish.

DEPRESSION PSYCHOSIS

This is too deep for me. I understand that the sheepish look fat boys often wear is symptomatic of depression psychosis.

They look sheepish because they know *you* know they aren't jolly.

This admission of weakness makes them feel sad. They realize they aren't up to snuff with their friends in the Elks Club.

Often this is the reason they are so boisterous. They try to out-talk, out-shout, out-dress others. It gives them a slight sense of superiority!

You usually find them off in a corner at the club

Elmer Organizes the F. B. I.

salving their spirits by munching a hamburger and washing it down with a short one.

Short one, is a quaint old term alluding to the now extinct 5¢ beer.

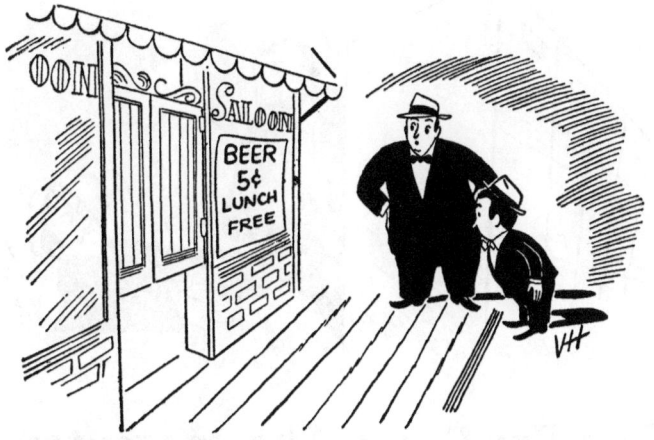

In fact, I believe fat boys need "speakeasies."

Places where they can congregate with the brethren to douse their sorrows in the forbidden calorie!

Places where they can play their favorite game, "Put On—Take Off."

FAT BOYS CAN'T CRAM FOR THE DOC'S EXAM—*Poor Elmer's Almanac.*

7

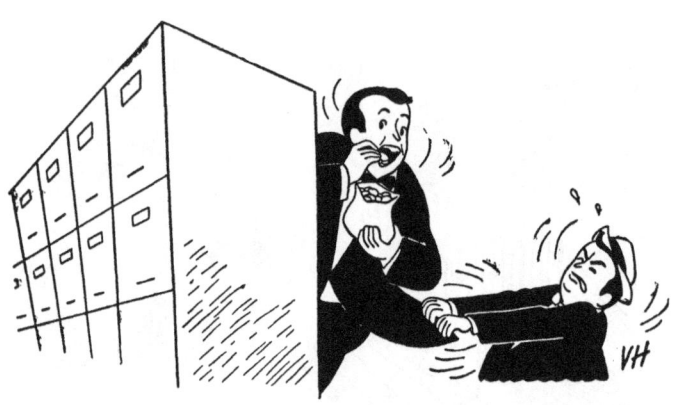

The Fat Boy's Thermometer Is Created

You know a fellow is getting fat when he looks more at his calorie card than the waitress.

I found, as the ex-fat boy, that if I was to continue to be the attraction in restaurants I'd better do some subtracting.

In the final days of King Elmer, the calorie hero,

The Fat Boy's Thermometer Is Created

headwaiters crowded around my table, not realizing that in feeding me they were killing their golden goose with their "house specialties."

One day I peeked into a full length mirror.

I was flabby-gasted.

Calories are nice little fellows to have around; but not around the waist line.

So right then and there I decided us fallen fat boys, members of our Fat Boys' Institute, needed a new and improved calorie counting card.

So the Fat Boy's Thermometer was created!

HOW THE THERMOMETER WORKS

Unlike our first calorie card, this one is designed mainly for fallen fat boys.

Of course, anyone taking the cure for the first time can use it.

And so also can fat boy's chubby mate or his tubby teenagers.

You place a clip at the starting point, and as you eat all day long, you keep sliding the clip up.

Since 1500 is top for any fatso on a Booster Course, that is the point where you find the *DANGER SIGNAL*.

So when you come to the fat boy's boiling point—*STOP!*

Now fatso who wants to go on an 1800 calorie spree just keeps on moving up.

The Fat Boy's Thermometer Is Created

And Slim Jim can eat until the mercury bubbles over the top.

It's all as simple as that!

IT'S MATHEMATICALLY SOUND

On back of The Fat Boy's Thermometer is a list of every-day foods old fatso consumes.

You won't find lobster Newburg or spaghetti Tetrazzini, because fatso on a diet better side-step these delectables, which put Diamond Jim Brady and Caruso in early graves.

You will find average foods—with average helpings.

When we speak of filets having 200 calories, that doesn't mean a side of cow.

It means a normal blue-plate size serving.

When you see vegetables at 50 calories, that means without a dosing in a lot of butter or margarine.

Remember, nothing you eat reduces you!

Even celery has a calorie or so.

HOW MANY CALORIES DO YOU NEED?

A good question.

You require fifteen calories, on the average, for every pound of weight if you are normal in height.

If you weigh 100 pounds you require fifteen times 100—or about 1500 calories.

Then you neither gain nor lose.

The Fat Boy's Thermometer Is Created

But in order to lose, you better cut down 500 or 1000 calories per day.

If you cut down 1000 calories that means ¼ lb., since there are 4000 calories to a pound.

If you want to gain—add a 1000 or more. Who cares?

If banquets or parties prevent the 1500 calories minimum per day, then go on a three-day spree. Set aside 4500 calories for three days.

Eat 'em all the first day—or divide them any way you want over the three days. That's up to you.

If you want to lose more than ¼ lb. per day—then see your doc!

That's up to him!

If you are real short, maybe 14 calories per pound is your requirement. If tall, 16 or 17 calories per pound. Fifteen, tho, is a good national average.

OUR F. B. I. HAS SOME SUCCESS

Ideas come flying into the F. B. I. from fallen fat boys who are taking the Booster Cure.

One tells about eating only stale bread, because then half the crumbs fall on the table.

Another keeps his belt tight, and he just can't stack in the wheat cakes without his belt sounding off, like a tight cinch on a quarter horse.

Sort of like an alarm in a chicken coop to warn you.

Another sends in this motto:

>Food that goes to waste certainly won't go to waist.

The Fat Boy's Thermometer Is Created

Perhaps the best of all came from a fellow in Seattle named Ernie who gave us our motto:

Eat tomorrow!

He says that since all fat boys always say, "I'll diet tomorrow," the slogan of our F. B. I. should be "Eat tomorrow!"

A neat idea! And so that's our slogan, "Eat tomorrow!"

I'M GETTING RID OF MY "PARTNER"

I was never a finicky eater. Ask Grandma Stroble. My type takes its pies, potatoes, and pot-pies as they come—and the devil take the hindmost.

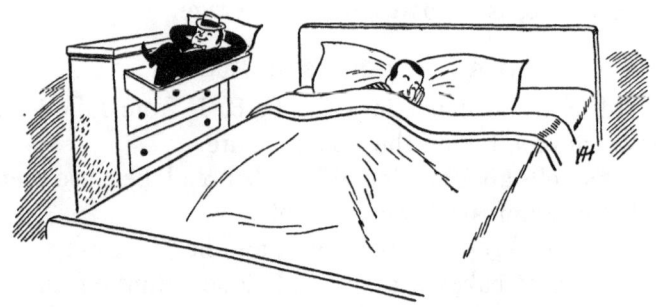

My "hindmost" certainly looked like the devil *had*. I'd again nearly become a food-fiend. A suet sucker. A calorie colossus. A carbarn for carbohydrates.

The Fat Boy's Thermometer Is Created

The chicken-pie-and-peach-cobbler lecture-circuit was to blame, until finally my lectures petered out. Who wanted to listen to a phony, anyway?

My "partner" was nearly back with me, that little fellow always sitting in a fat boy's lap.

But the F. B. I. saved me. It came just in time. My weight has gone down four pounds! I'm on the bright side again. I no longer need a double bed all to myself.

A GOOD PHILOSOPHY

Us fallen fat boys, fugitives from girth, soon make a lot of interesting discoveries.

For example, it isn't what you eat *first* that puts on weight, but what you eat *last*.

That is, the last few things you should'a' saved for dawn—tomorrow!

Often we actually go on a potato binge, a spaghetti or candy spree.

We just get so doggone hungry for starch or sweets, we dunk ourselves in it.

But being good and faithful members, we record each binge on our Fat Boy's Thermometer (as long as the chart holds out), then make amends the next few days.

So that during a week's time we haven't gone too far overboard.

But we do it out in the open. We don't sneak our sins no more.

The Fat Boy's Thermometer Is Created

We realize it is all right to eat so-called fattening dishes, creamed soups, Newburgs, peanuts, doughnuts. Just so long as we don't do the job all up at the same meal. So long as for the day we don't total over 1500 calories.

And boy, when the Booster Cure is over—we can go back to 2500 calories per day, and not gain an ounce!

IT'S KNOWLEDGE, NOT LUCK

Losing weight is not luck—it's knowledge.

If you can count up to 1500, you can not gain weight.

We learned, too, that five small-size dinners put on less weight than one gigantic dinner.

When you overeat the stomach stretches way out of proportion, like a balloon. Then, as it shrinks back, it sets up a disturbance known as "hunger pains."

But with three or five small-size meals, the stomach never stretches out of proportion, and you seldom get hunger pains.

Remember, too, "after seven days your stomach shrinks in many ways," and you won't feel hungry.

Often you gain weight to start with, since the fat, in losing nourishment, gets spongy and absorbs water—and water weighs more than food.

But inside of seven or ten days, the water gets pretty heavy for your lard, which drops it all of a sudden like a hot check.

The Fat Boy's Thermometer Is Created

WHAT IS A CALORIE?

Calories are units of energy in food. They're the tiny hunks of coal the body burns to keep going.

You burn up 1800 calories every day just breathing and moving around normally. The more you move, the more you work, the more you burn up.

Housewives can burn up 2100 to 3000. Office workers about the same. Laborers and "gossips" can go as high as 4000 calories a day! Bookworms about 1900.

Dump in more coal than you burn—and the rest stores up in the form of fat.

The reason why two people can eat the same things, yet one gains and the other loses, is that the loser has his "motor" running faster.

Put 20 gallons of gas into two Ford cars. But set the motor of one car running faster, and it burns up the 20 gallons sooner than the slow-running car.

Which is why your wife, jumping around all day, tapping her fingers, talking with her hands, feet, and mouth all at the same time, remains skinny.

And *you* stack on the heft!

DID YOU KNOW THIS?

That an average family of four eats two and a half tons of food per year, and that includes:

690 lbs. of potatoes
12 cans of sauerkraut

The Fat Boy's Thermometer Is Created

    15 baskets of tomatoes
  350 lbs. of sugar
  698 quarts of milk
  131 dozen eggs

Which is why, with a knowledge of this, the class yell of the Fat Boys' Institute, from this day on, becomes:

> Less on the fork, and more on the plate;
> That's our big secret of losing weight!

REMEMBER: EAT TOMORROW!—*Poor Elmer's Almanac.*

8

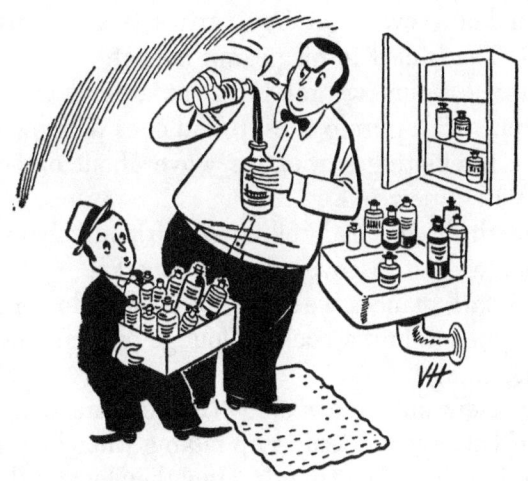

Some Startling Bulge-Banishing Facts

As I told you in *The Fat Boy's Book*, and, as I lose weight the second time I'm finding out again, there are real handicaps to losing weight.

Outside of seats getting harder quicker, and you get-

Some Startling Bulge-Banishing Facts

ting cold faster nights, you lose contact with fat boy sociability.

Were you to ask me my greatest loss, outside of lard, I'd say the pleasure of discussing burp pills.

You know every fat boy carries them in his burp pocket. That's next to his peanut pocket.

Ah! the hours we fat boys sat around comparing green pills with purple ones; round ones with oval ones.

The fascinating stories we wove about our experiences with a new pill.

The thrills we had telling our friends about some new one we just discovered on the market.

The dark glances we'd get from some doctor friend who happened into a cocktail lounge or gym where we fat ones hung out.

He knew only too well what we were discussing. For we'd always suddenly stop talking when he came in.

But our drugstore friends. How they loved us! Every birthday, the one at the corner always sent me a remembrance—and a new circular.

I sure miss Joe's remembrances.

THEN CAME THE F. B. I.

Now we have as great a thrill discussing newest weight-reducing methods. Not burp medicines. But methods this time.

I can remember when old George read up and found some facts about Bacchus.

Some Startling Bulge-Banishing Facts

For example, did you know that the old theory that water drunk the morning after will start you all over again after a night with Bacchus is bunk?

T'aint so. Ask your doc.

And did you know that, scientifically, a hang-over is alcoholic action on the nerves "due to lack of sufficient oxygen"? Which is why a sudden breath of air when you come out of the club's cellar often makes you see two moons!

How wonderful backyards look around 11 P.M.!

This same F. B. I. researcher came up with the fact that milk, ice cream, or olive oil before a round with Bacchus slows up the time this man with the grapevine headgear takes over.

Wow! When the stuff wears off, though, you get a double wallop!

That if you take three—not two—aspirins before retiring, if you can find your mouth, the chances of a headache for breakfast are remote!

And lastly he exploded the theory that whiskey is good for snake bites.

It isn't.

It seems alcohol and snake venom *both* lower metabolism, and both working at the same time are dangerous!

So take your snake bites and liquor separately if you want to be a member in good standing of the F. B. I.

Some Startling Bulge-Banishing Facts

WE WORK UP A GOOD ONE HERE

While humor helps us over a tough job, yet behind the humor, or with it, or around it, is a lot of common sense.

For example, one fat boy came rushing into our Sizzle Lab in Dallas where we often meet, with a real tummy-trimming idea.

The 3-B's Method of losing fat.

Boil! Broil! and Bake!

If you sell this idea to the cook, if you edit each restaurant menu to eliminate fried foods, you can eat nearly twice as much.

Take an egg for example. It is 65 when boiled—and up to 120 when fried!

If you broil that pork chop, it has some 50 calories less than when you pan-fry it and let the fat of the rind ooze into the lean meat!

You'll find the 3 B's carved in many a fat boy's kitchen table these days. That is, if he is a member of the Fat Boys' Institute and carries his pocket calorie card, The Fat Boy's Thermometer.

DON'T ELIMINATE ALL FOODS

Remember the psychology of the F. B. I. is to tell fat folks, "Yes—you can eat!" instead of "No—you can't!"

If you look hard enough you'll find foods you can eat and still lose weight.

Some Startling Bulge-Banishing Facts

For example, you can eat around four lobsters to one fried pork chop—that is, if you *can* eat four of them.

Naturally the amount of butter on the lobster has something to do with it.

You not only can—but MUST—eat some starch daily.

Starch is needed to burn up calories. It sets fire to protein.

So don't begrudge yourself a little spaghetti, or a spud, or bread—just don't go overboard and entertain all three at the same setting!

Edit your food wisely, and you can even have your cake—and not feel it!

A WORD ON SEX

No particular foods enhance your sex vigor, as one of our more ribald agents found.

All you need to keep in proper shape is the proper combination of all foods, Agent X reported.

Fat does reduce pep though.

That is why you see a spry fox terrier doing all the barking, as he runs circles around a St. Bernard.

This applies to humans as well!

Overeating won't help your vigor or pep. You can't store up sex.

But if you get on too strict a diet you'll lose interest in high streetcar steps on windy days.

Some Startling Bulge-Banishing Facts

HOW ABOUT VITAMIN AND MINERAL PILLS?

Let me start by saying, "We take them—all the time!" —but particularly when we are trying to lose weight.

It stands to reason that less food means less calories —and less vitamins and minerals too!

That's why you cannot rely on a low-calory diet to give your body all the vitamins and minerals it needs to stay healthy.

You've got to rely on a good supplement—one that supplies good quantities of *all* the essential vitamins and minerals.

They have practically no caloric value. You'd have to eat thousands of calories worth of food to obtain the vitamins and minerals you get from one calory-free pill.

They help eliminate hidden hunger—actually reduce your appetite!

People on a reducing diet who take 'em generally look better, feel better, have more pep and energy.

The F. B. I. therefore recommends a vitamin-mineral supplement as a "must."

VITAMINS DO HELP YOU

The deeper the tan—the less D you'll absorb. (*Hope Miami doesn't ban this book. Wouldn't mind if Boston did, though.*)

Drugstore vitamins are as good for you as those you get from the garden.

Some Startling Bulge-Banishing Facts

Deep green and yellow colors in vegetables indicate lots of vitamins are present.

Baking soda used in cooking kills off many of the vitamins.

So does overcooking, or too much water.

Avoid stirring, as vitamins will evaporate from the pot.

As leafy vegetables wilt, the vitamin content is destroyed.

Plunge frozen foods quickly into hot water—to preserve the vitamins in cooking. If left to defrost gradually, they'll lose their vitamins.

WHAT VITAMINS DO

Vitamins are an excellent supplement to dieting.

When you cut down on food, you also cut your vitamin intake.

Vitamin pills will keep you fit during the skirmish with your spare tire.

Vitamin A is good for the eyes or skin. Liver, butter, eggs are loaded with it. Also beets or any yellow plant such as carrots.

The B vitamins are essential to practically every function of your body and glands. Deficiency can cause anything from frazzled nerves and fatigue to constipation, anemia, headaches, and skin disorders. The B vitamins are found in whole grain breads, meat, fish, green vegetables.

Some Startling Bulge-Banishing Facts

Vitamin C is necessary to healthy teeth and gums, blood vessels, glands. Deficiency can cause bleeding gums, tooth decay, varicose veins, lowered resistance to infection, slow wound healing. You will find it in oranges and other citrus fruits—also in cabbage. Cooking destroys Vitamin C. So eat your fruits and vegetables raw whenever possible.

Vitamin D is necessary to good teeth and bones. Your body cannot make use of calcium and phosphorus unless Vitamin D is present. You get it from sunshine, from irradiated milk and from fish liver oils. Ordinary foods furnish very little Vitamin D.

WHAT MINERALS DO

Iron is necessary to healthy red blood. Without iron, blood cannot carry oxygen to the cells. Deficiency can cause nutritional anemia resulting in a tired, run-down feeling. Iron deficiency is particularly common to people who spend most of their time indoors—particularly common to the female sex. You will find iron in green leafy vegetables, meat, fish.

Calcium and phosphorus are needed for healthy teeth, bones, muscles and blood. Deficiency may result in brittle bones, tooth decay, muscle soreness and spasm. These minerals are found in milk, cream, cheese and eggs.

Naturally the above represents only a small part of all the information about vitamins and minerals and

Some Startling Bulge-Banishing Facts

what they do. However, it should give you some idea of their importance to your health.

Remember this F. B. I. basic rule for good health—*while* taking it off and *after* taking it off eat a low-calorie vitamin-rich diet and be sure to take a good vitamin-mineral supplement along with it!

WHEN IS A FAT BOY FAT?

Editorials have been written in such papers as the Chicago *News* and the Kansas City *Star* by writers who ask, "When is a fat boy fat?"

When do you sit back and say, "It is about time I take Elmer's Calorie Cure"?

Mine came, as you know, when I whistled for the dog and my wife laughed. The dog was under me all the time.

When she presented me with a walking-stick to "press door bells."

I suddenly realized I was fat, too, when she ordered in twin beds, asking me did I look at myself lately, *sidewise!*

Then is when I said to myself, "You are a Big Blimp Boy, Elmer."

When that day comes in your life, you'll know it—just as you know love when it finally comes around.

PANGS OF HUNGER ARE BETTER THAN PANGS OF REMORSE—
Poor Elmer's Almanac.

9

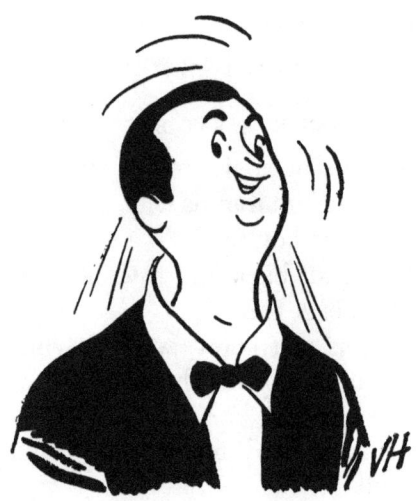

Even the Small Fry Tell Elmer Off

Now it is one thing when the wife takes a retake on your tummy profile.

Another when the doc shakes his head, and the undertaker tips his hat. You can slough that off too.

Even the Small Fry Tell Elmer Off

But when your own child comes up and starts giving you advice on how to shed suet, then you begin to realize you have slipped off the wagon.

"Hey, Pop," says our little Linda Beth, "my school teacher read your book, lost a sack of sass and suet, and now is reading the diet act to us kids."

I smile with great pride until she adds:

"But how come, Pop, you ain't practicing what you preach? How come you *say* eat spinach but we catch you *eating* peanut brittle?"

I hang my bags low on my eyes.

"How come you let the bay window get back into the act? Us kids down at school were using you as a shining example for our own lives."

She sighs. I sigh. As she says:

"You were just about to replace Hopalong Cassidy in popularity, but ah now!" She shakes her head.

"You are being branded a medical fake . . . a local freak . . . a neighborhood jerk!"

I GET TOLD OFF

So the little gal tells off her old man, and really comes forth with some small fry and teenage fat-boy hints, which make me more determined than ever to get down nearer to Hopalong's size.

"Us kids," says Linda Beth, "began to realize even we can get unnecessarily fat for fun. Why, Roger got so

Even the Small Fry Tell Elmer Off

he could almost roll down the street. He never made the ball team."

She shakes her head, "But his mom gives him your book. Then Fatty Rogers, as we called him, slimmed off 15 lbs. of hot dawgs and milk shakes that had made him a softie."

I sigh. She sighs. "And now Thin Boy Rogers, him, imagine, is on the school team . . . golly gosh, and does he look tall and handsome once more."

I turn red in the face when I realize how many hot dawgs and how much popcorn I had just that afternoon at the ball park!

SMALL FRY KEEPS UP THE NEEDLE

"Then there was Jennie—a first grade fatso of the teens—our class wallflower. Never got a date to any class picnic. Even had to carry her own books back and forth to Junior High.

"But then, Pops, she borrows that book of yours from Thin Boy Rogers, who doesn't need it any longer, and today even teacher remarked how pretty she was, minus a chubby backside that really stood out when she rode on her bicycle."

She needles me on even harder.

"But, Pop, watcha think—who do you suppose is now carrying her books and buying her choc sodas? Why Thin Boy Rogers—gee, you sure did a good thing for us kids and teenagers."

Then she slumped over a Mexican-style chair in my

Even the Small Fry Tell Elmer Off

den. Grunting to herself, "But it's all over. No more am I a Hero's Daughter. I'm a Freud's Fraud!"

I wish I were dead!

SO ELMER GETS MADDER

I get madder by the minute, or should I say pound?

I'm more determined than ever now to whittle the bay window back to man size, that is, one-man size.

I read up and find a lot of information for small fry and teenagers to use, if I could again get them believing in Hopalong Elmer. Gosh, if I could only earn that title —Hopalong Elmer!

For example, I'd show them some real new calorie info such as: an avocado is nearly ten times as fattening as a tomato.

I'd tell 'em, too, that when they munch on a fig it has as many calories as a whole bunch of grapes . . . that even an onion has 50 calories, and a garlic clove has 2 of them hidden in the aroma.

Yep, think Old Hopalong Elmer, the Kalorie Kid, will thin down and help children.

ELMER SETS THE F.B.I. ON THE TRAIL

So I call in the Charter Members of my newly formed F.B.I., the Fat Boys' Institute.

I tell them to help kids keep the proper weight, that is, gain if they need; slice off if they have something extra.

Even the Small Fry Tell Elmer Off

That proper weight makes play more fun, gets them better marks in school because they aren't drowsy from too much food, and they won't be wallflowers any more.

That the pudgy small fry is not at all happy, might even get a neurosis, if he turns around when somebody yells, "Hey, fattie!"

Yet they can gain weight—or lose it—if they knew such simple kid-eating facts as:

> Popcorn has 100 calories; a hot dog, ball park size, has 300; most small soft drinks have 65 calories, and the larger ones around 120.
>
> That buttermilk has half as many calories as sweet milk, and cottage cheese sure fills you up but keeps you thinned down.

So the F.B.I. goes to work for kids.

SOME MORE INTERESTING FACTS

First, our F.B.I. found that it is better for small fry to be a little overweight than underweight. It is better to be husky than spindly.

But a "little overweight" doesn't mean looking like a small-size pickle barrel, for that's way too much size for fun.

We learned that small fry are often fat because they imitate the eating habits of their parents, and if Pop guzzles six bowls of soup and sops gravy up with five slices of bread, so will small fry.

Little Wilbur is often satisfied with half a cantaloupe

Even the Small Fry Tell Elmer Off

until he sees Mom eat three hunks of her best chocolate cake, smothered in ice cream and with nuts on top.

Now we issue one warning: *no food is to be eliminated.*

Just don't mix them hit and miss. I mean, eat your macaroni, but not at a meal where you also have potatoes and gravy all over the plate.

Have a doughnut on and off, but not just ahead of green-apple pie. Eat a bag of peanuts and some hot dawgs, but then don't expect to munch half a pound of taffy candy.

Take anything you want—but in turn, one at a time!

Each is swell in its place—but keep them in their place.

Don't mix foods hit-and-miss.

FOODS THAT REALLY HELP KIDS

Small fry and their teen-age "elders" can easily learn that certain foods do certain things to their growing bodies. For example:

Fat-Boy Growing Foods. They are the meats, fish, potatoes, cereals, cheeses, milk. They have the right vitamins and minerals to help the bones grow and to give muscles.

Fat-Boy Health Foods. These foods have lots of vitamins, such as A, which combats the colds in the head that upset studies and spoil games. So eat lots of cottage cheese, tomato juice, orange juice, most other

Even the Small Fry Tell Elmer Off

fruits, peanut butter sandwiches, and butter, which is loaded with A.

Fat-Boy School Foods. Doctors call them "brain foods," for they help girls and boys develop their "thinking ability." Such as celery, fish, and always, of course, lots of milk and cottage cheese, which is a milk product.

Fat-Boy Energy Foods. Girls and boys who are active need candy, soft drinks, anything with sugar in it to give a quick lift. Spaghetti and macaroni have starch that gives us "action." They need chocolate milk shakes —but of course, not too much of the sweets, especially for those who are overweight.

Fat-Boy Thinning Foods. Meat, fish, cottage cheese, Ry-Krisp, fruits galore, salads, cabbage, any vegetables except dried ones such as lima beans, and be sure to trim the fat off the meat. Buttermilk instead of sweet milk.

Fat-Boy Fattening Foods. Sweet milk instead of buttermilk. Lots of peanut butter between thick slices of bread. Pork and beans. Ice cream galore—and put on thick chocolate sauces and peanuts. Potatoes with lots of gravy, and avocado salads and thick creamed soups.

It's all in knowing what to eat!

HEALTH BEGINS WITH SMALL FRY

We aren't born to like certain foods; we learn to like them by seeing what our elders like and eat.

Only temper is inherited. Not food likes.

Even the Small Fry Tell Elmer Off

So Dad and Mom should set a good example for small fry.

Small fry can just as easily learn to like cabbage salad as creamed asparagus or lentil soup.

Nothing is funnier, remember, than a fatso child wobbling along, trying to catch a fast ball, to skip rope, roller skate, or ride a bicycle.

Nothing is more pitiful than a teen-ager on the wallflower line, watching others have fun dancing.

Yet it is easy for small fry to slice off fat by watching Kid Kalorie just as his parents should do.

For example, small fry should realize custard pie is just half as fattening as most other pies such as green apple loaded with sugar to remove the "green."

That lima beans have 200 calories per cup—yet most other vegetables have only 50 calories.

That rhubarb per cup is 200 calories, same as a doughnut and more than a glass of sweet milk. That brick ice cream has less calories than hand-packed because in hand packing you force out all the air.

That cabbage salads have around 25 calories, while salads with roquefort dressing can go as high as 200 calories.

The first ten years of "eating habits" make or break small fry.

LITTLE KNOWN FACTS ON EATING

Even the manufacturers guard against their customers' eating too much of anything, since if you overeat

Even the Small Fry Tell Elmer Off

on an item you skip it for days and days, often weeks, you are so satiated with it.

So they will tell you to eat peanut butter on and off, and don't overdose on soft drinks, candy bars, cookies and cakes.

Eat your bread with butter or margarine. But treat butter and margarine kindly. Don't use it like Pop does axle grease on that old gas buggy of his.

And when you plan to go to a birthday party, go light on food before the party; and at the party, settle for one small-fry-size cake and ice cream. No manufacturer wants you to have the tummy ache and quit his product for a year or so.

Broil the 'burger. It tastes better. Has half the calories it would if fried. And when the turkey comes around, eat the white meat; it has less calories than the dark.

Besides, Pop likes the dark!

Say kids, this is Okay Stuff, isn't it?

Maybe Linda Beth now won't think so harsh of her Dad, and her teacher won't sniff her nose and call him "phony."

Maybe I'll still be called Hopalong Elmer.

Gosh, imagine me on a stone horse in the park!

SHE'S LOST HER WEIGHT;
SHE'S GOT HER FIRST DATE!
—*Poor Elmer's Almanac.*

10

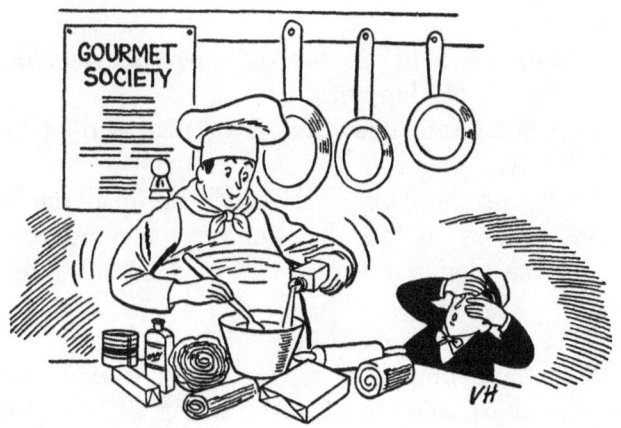

How Elmer Spots an F.B.I. Recruit

It takes a crook to catch a crook, a fat boy to catch another.

We of the F. B. I. can always spot a "first timer," or for that matter a fat boy who's already done a stretch or two up the River of Diet.

How Elmer Spots an F. B. I. Recruit

A fallen fat boy, especially, always aims his derrière at the softest chair in the room.

Down pillows are his delight—and downfall.

He seldom stands at a bar. Too much work. He goes for the plush lounge seats, in the darkest part of the joint.

"Pursuit of food" to the old-timer is synonymous with "Pursuit of Happiness."

He's first in any chow line. Lead man at the table—last to leave.

He figures the skinny fellows will eat up all the food before he gets to it if he saunters too nonchalantly toward the food, pretending the food doesn't interest him.

Thus, fat begets more fat.

Swimming burns up most calories; running next; walking third; standing fourth; sitting fifth; sleeping sixth.

Where do you find fat boys—sixth, of course!

ALL THE SAME TRIBE

Likes join likes. We of the fallen fat boys' society are sort of like evangelists.

We're trying to redeem ourselves and others for past overeating sins.

Our job is saving seats—not souls.

At the altar of obesity we've dedicated ourselves to the banishing of our bay windows.

How Elmer Spots an F. B. I. Recruit

If you are one of those perennial fatsos, man, woman, or child, who have dieted, bragged, relaxed and gained it all back—you, too, can be saved.

You don't need a tambourine. Just the Fat Boy's Thermometer, and the education to count up to 1500.

It isn't WHAT you eat so much as how much of the wrong foods you shove in.

Some grub you can gorge on, like sauerkraut, pickles, cottage cheese, and cole slaw; with other foods, a little goes a long way, calorie-wise.

Which is why we say knowledge can save your seats!

EMBARRASSING MOMENTS FOR FATSO

Being a fat boy often brings on an inferiority complex. He can't dance like he wants. He huffs and puffs in the arms of his mate, or sweats too much.

He has embarrassing moments, such as the times he is caught eating two pieces of apple pie.

My most embarrassing moment happened in Tampa.

I visited Ybor City, down Tampa way, with friend Tony Florez.

While he shoved factory-fresh Berings toward my mouth, Columbia Restaurant's Spanish waiters moved appetizing yellow rice and chicken toward my tummy.

I enjoyed both. I had to. I hate to disappoint a client.

How Elmer Spots an F. B. I. Recruit

Tony beamed. Joe Fernandez, the headwaiter, beamed. Customers around us beamed.

I burped!

THE FIVE-POUND SYSTEM

Things are different now.

No longer do I need to consume 1500 calories. My weight is again about normal, and soon I'll be back to 2500 calories.

If I work late—work harder—mow the lawn, or fail to get my full eight hours, I might even get up to 3000 calories.

In fact, my metabolism is gaining strength again, and will protect me, if I do overeat now and then, by snapping me back.

But us F. B. I. boys now have a "Warning Device."

It's a good old scale!

After we are down to our desired weight, say 185 (where I am again headed for), and the scale pops up to 190—I watch out for a few days.

I pull myself down a few days to 1500-calorie eating!

That's a mighty good thing to have around the bathroom—a scale.

Use it every morning, and when it creeps up five pounds—then let that be the Warning!

Boy, for a scale that would ring a bell when we weigh too much!

How Elmer Spots an F. B. I. Recruit

Slow up for the next three days—and you'll never again be a fallen fat boy!

WHY WEIGHT VARIES EACH DAY

Some folks are real lucky. Their thermostat—their metabolism—takes care of them perfectly.

They have learned, through instinct or just luck, how much to eat daily so that they never "gain or lose in 20 years."

If they weighed each day, though, they'd learn a lot.

For example, after a night of Bacchus you are apt to have a lot of water content for the next two days. Water absorbed by the fat.

It soon breathes away or otherwise disappears.

On damp, rainy days you're apt to weigh more since you don't let off enough moisture.

Cheer up, the first dry day and you'll dehydrate.

Which is why weighing once a week is good enough!

HOW TO BEAT OLD DEVIL HUNGER

If it weren't for so-called "hunger pains," the contraction of the stomach walls yelping for more food, many a fat boy would be a thin boy.

Some foods—the kind fat boys are usually fondest of —keep the stomach beefing. Keep it howling for more.

That is why fatso gives up reducing, and becomes a backslider.

How Elmer Spots an F. B. I. Recruit

For example, banana splits. Or chocolate sodas—the plump gal's folly—are only temporarily satisfying.

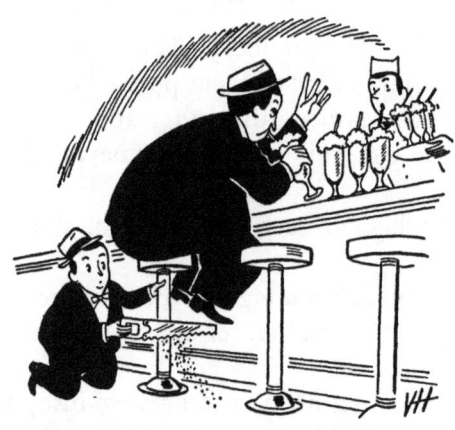

In short order they leave the stomach—and it is ready for another short order of 500 or so calories.

But proteins—meats, fish, cheese—stay a long time in the stomach being digested. They don't leave you hungry.

They seem to fill fat boy's hollow leg, and stay put until the next authorized meal.

Pulling the belt tighter often cramps the stomach walls so they can't contract and make you hungry.

Any hobo knows that!

How Elmer Spots an F. B. I. Recruit

WHAT ABOUT CIGARETTE SMOKING?

This is Number One Question on a fallen fat boy's list.

Our Research Division really went into this to help the backsliders.

We learned the true facts.

Is cigarette smoking harmful or not? We don't get into this! We just know smoking will hold the weight down.

Many a fat boy has GAINED up to 20 pounds when he stopped smoking.

The reason being that inhaling does tickle the metabolism into slight action.

You do get the lift they advertise, and this small lift several times a day burns up a few calories that otherwise would rest in peace under the second chin.

This is true with cigar and pipe smokers.

Then, too, when a cigarette is in your hand it can't hold a sweet Lady Finger.

Since taste is often 50 per cent smell, according to taste experts, when you smoke you dull the sensitive nose buds. You can't smell well, so when Aunt Emmy puts on a pork roast you don't drool so fast and so often.

F.B.I. FACTS ON ALCOHOL

Several doctor members of our F.B.I., experts on metabolic ailments, came up with interesting reasons why alcohol makes you eat more.

How Elmer Spots an F. B. I. Recruit

You'd think alcohol stimulated your appetite. It doesn't. It *dulls* the "food senses," and they don't respond and tell you that you are full up and should stop eating.

So with no warning from the tummy, you keep right on eating. Like filling your gas tank without a dash board indicator. You never know when the tank is filled up until it floods over the fender.

Alcohol taken in excess, however, authorities point out, works in reverse. It takes away all desire for food. If you step up to the lunch counter with a couple under your belt, you are apt to overeat. But if you step up with a dozen (if you can still step), you are apt to find no inner urge to eat anything. Alcoholics go days without food.

The learned docs in their F.B.I. confab brought out another interesting fact: why alcohol removes worry. Again it is a case of dulling, not stimulating, the nerves. Dulled nerves aren't so acute to your thoughts and worries, and so you raise your heels and say, "Wot the heck—so the house burned down, I lost my money, and my wife left home! Yippee!!"

THREE TYPES OF FALLEN FATSOS

At this stage of our F. B. I. research we are able to classify various types of perennial fat boys.

Scientifically, they are:

How Elmer Spots an F. B. I. Recruit

1. *The Lazy Type.* He gets his fat back on because, once lost, the thrill of showing off his bragging belt is over with. He becomes lazy with food. Lazy with activity.

He's just fat 'cause he puts in more than he gives out.

A horse that eats too many oats never leaves the stable.

The same with a fat boy. He never leaves his home!

2. *The Glandular.* Not you, bub. For only one in every 10,000 fat cases is glandular. The glands are just double-crossed, and this is the only time where it is true, "Everything I eat turns to fat."
3. *The Psychic.* He is bored with life. Eats to overcome boredom. He is lonesome; eats to have something to do. He has home or financial troubles; eats to forget them.

Here, at last, is the fat boy for the couch consultant! He's in grave need of a sofa session!

But again you can sum up all excess fat to one thing. *Only food puts on weight.* Not air. Not water. *Just food.* That is, too much of the wrong food.

If you eat more than you put out, you'll gain.

BE SURE INTAKE EQUALS OUTPUT—*Poor Elmer's Almanac.*

11

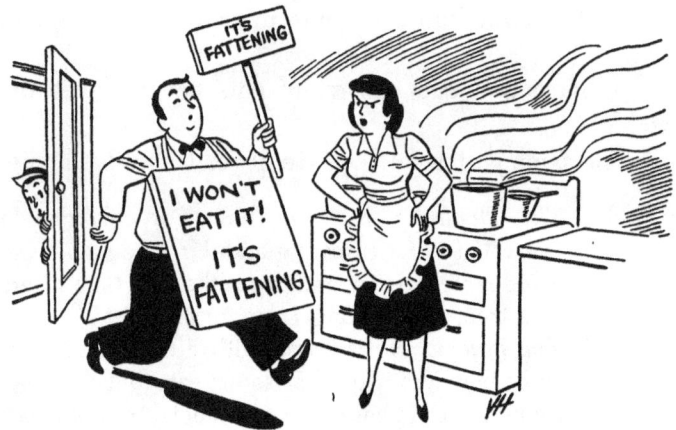

Calorie Loses Fat Boy

Plots of most plays and stories follow this formula: Boy meets girl, boy loses girl, boy gets girl back.

The story of the average fat boy is the same, we of The Fat Boys' Institute agree.

Calorie catches fat boy, calorie loses fat boy, calorie gets fat boy back.

Calories have captured us F. B. I. fellows again—but not for long.

Calorie Loses Fat Boy

Our Booster Cure for fallen fat boys who have backslid into their downfall is beginning to shuck their surplus suet.

Soon the pendulum will swing back.

Once more it will be, "Calorie loses fat boy!"

The quicker the better. I'm tired of leading a double life!

Me and my partner are about to separate, little Kid Kalorie sitting so long in my lap!

INSPIRATION FROM "WEIGHTY" SAYINGS

While speaking for my supper in hotels across the country, I learned that the American public's pulse quickens when you mention sex, TV, or who is President and why.

Now I add "diet" to the list of scintillating conversation-makers.

Mention diet and everyone perks up.

This is because nobody figures his or her weight is "just right." As we say in *Poor Elmer's Almanac:*

> There's no such thing as the normal guy;
> Your weight's too low or else too high.

Even a 90-pound secretary thinks she'd be more "perfect" at 96—or 102.

Discovering this situation made me philosophical, for after all aren't all fat boys philosophical?

Having reduced once, I used to sit back, fire up a

Calorie Loses Fat Boy

Corral, Wodiska y Cia special and mentally rove through *Poor Elmer's Almanac*.

My homemade jingles still apply:

> Food that's fried is tough on the hide.
> MORAL: People who keep their mouths closed never gain weight.
> Bread is better toasted; meat better roasted.
> If you're slight—get an appetite.
> It isn't fate that puts on weight.
> Be shrewd—edit your food.
> People who edit will never regret it.

But when I again became a fat boy, a backslider, I went into some deeper stuff, as we always do when death faces us.

I started looking up the real intellectual heavyweights on weight fast-talk.

ELMER GETS "LEARNED"

I quote from a fellow named Franklin, to wit:

> To lengthen thy life, lessen thy meals.

In plain language, he means "eat less—live longer." He also said:

> I saw a few die of hunger; of eating, a hundred thousand.

Calorie Loses Fat Boy

Same stuff, only in more fancy language. It means folks don't die in bread lines, only at Smörgåsbords.

A fellow named Tom Jefferson made this contribution to fat-boy philosophy:

> We never repent of having eaten too little.

Such sayings, of course, to us F. B. I. members are ABC.

And then there was Hippocrates who quipped:

> Fat men are more likely to die suddenly than slender.

A modern doc, member of our overweight fraternity, puts it this way:

> The skinny rats bury the fat ones.

Sort of like his words better, don't you? More to the point.

EVEN THE ARABS HELP ELMER

I like some of those Arab and Spanish proverbs such as:

> In a well-provided house, supper is soon served.

All fat boys say "Amen" to that.
Also to:

> There's no accounting for taste.

Calorie Loses Fat Boy

and

Suppers have killed more than Avicenna cured.

Arthur Brisbane put it this way:

You eat yourself to the grave with your teeth.

Or:

Half of what you eat keeps you alive—the other half kills you.

But perhaps the most potent of all sayings is the one:

Pleasures pass—but sorrows stay on!

How true, how true! As many an overeating fat boy has said *after* the banquet!

FAT-BOY PIPE DREAMS

The banker dreams of making a million; the shoe clerk of marrying the boss's daughter.

The fat boy dreams of food.

Cherries jubilee, Thousand Island dressing, shrimp Arno, sweet-and-sour spareribs—anything that is calorie packed.

They forget the advice of a fellow named Bill Penn:

If thou rise with an appetite, thou art sure never to sit down without one.

Calorie Loses Fat Boy

Fat boys are fond of torturing themselves, which is why they have their downfalls. Deliberately they stand in front of a Child's window and drool over somebody making flapjacks or frying ham and eggs.

Self-torture!

So our F. B. I. has this motto hanging over our nibble table:

> Talk that's centered on sugar and starches,
> Soon will bear down on your arches!

Instead of gabbing about food, we get into an argument now on what some President said to a general! We soon lose our appetites!

OUR F. B. I. BATTLES IGNORANCE

Eating a meal without knowing the food facts is like buying a pig-in-a-poke.

That is one reason why fat boys who have lost 10, 20, or 40 pounds during the summer gain it all back during the winter.

You don't know what you'll wind up with.

For example, our Research Division learned that starches are busted apart by the saliva in our mouths, so we eat them slowly.

Meats, on the other hand, are mostly digested in the stomach, and from there on.

We learned a great scientific fact that gave us our Fat-Boy Coat of Arms:

Calorie Loses Fat Boy

That salesmen and reporters, being only mildly active, outlive wrestlers, gin rummy players, lawn mowers, tennis players, and golfers.

This is an exact medical fact. So our group quickly decided our emblem, our symbol, our coat of arms MUST be: The Hammock!

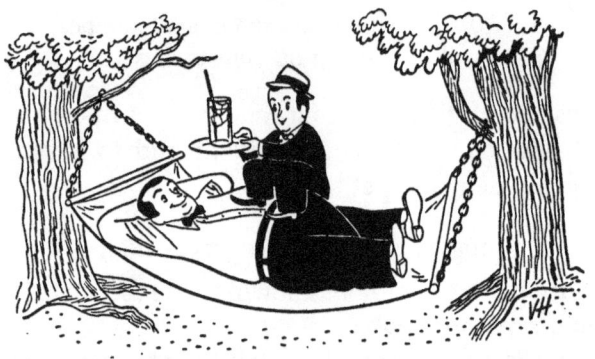

No one was ever reported dying in The Hammock!

A REPORT FROM THE SAFETY BOYS

That part of the government that goes in for safety figures and records, makes an interesting discovery:

> Accidents are more prevalent among overweights than slim folks.

This is due to the fact that the bigger you get, the slower you move.

Calorie Loses Fat Boy

Your reflexes are slower than the machine's knife coming down at you in a factory; slower than the car in the hands of a juvenile.

You may have a sturdy stomach in your thirties, but a car in its sixties will get you!

Of course, the fact that fat folks daydream a lot about their meals might also be a factor contributing to their great accident record!

A blonde in the eye got one of our new members the other day before he was sufficiently innoculated.

That is, the blonde was in his eye while a fender was in the six inches of fat which up till that moment he liked to sit on!

IGNORANCE AIN'T BLISS

If all fat boys knew such facts, they'd ask help from a skinny fellow when they crossed the streets.

They'd realize that when they are full of food, they are relaxed, have less muscular energy, are less alert, and as a drunk needs support—so do they.

It's funny—fat boys know the ingredients of a Mohido or a Zombie, but ask them if an orange juice or spinach contains Vitamin B and they'll give you a dumb stare.

They'd know that Vitamin B is killed by the first sip of alcohol, and that next day they should eat up on cabbage, whole wheat germ, and a Vitamin B pill or two.

Calorie Loses Fat Boy

That salads too long soaked lose their vitamin content in the water—that foods cooked fast retain more vitamins than those cooked at a slow boil.

Soak fast. Cook fast. Two good rules for fat boy's kitchen!

If wives of fat boys would only learn how to kill the calorie in the kitchen, instead of the vitamin, their mates would be in better shape!

They'd know, too, that food "under glass" would keep their mates from being "two time losers."

As long as it STAYS under glass.

(Elmer's back down to 190!)

GET UP FROM THE TABLE AND LEAVE IT FLAT;
THAT'S ELMER'S SECRET OF PREVENTING FAT.
—Poor Elmer's Almanac.

12

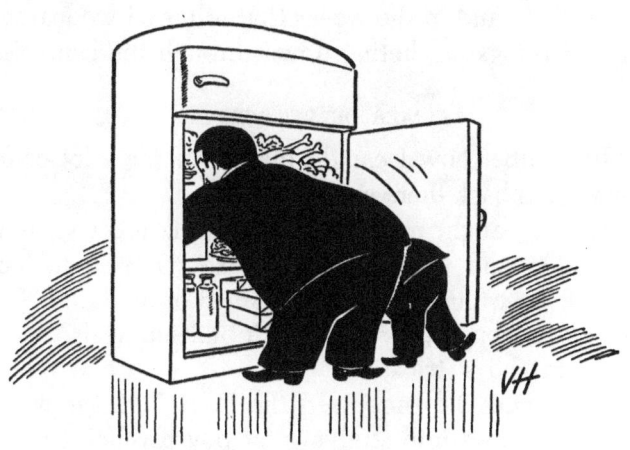

Little Known Facts on Fat Boys

Lots of folks say the sole reason some people get fat is psychological.

They say it's all in your head.

Okay, then—don't be a fathead. *Think thin.*

When I went from my famous 230 pounds down to

Little Known Facts on Fat Boys

186, I even lost one quarter size in my hat size—so it's true that fat boys *can* be fatheads.

What are other dieting facts little known to fat boys? I brought this subject up at a weighty meeting of our F. B. I., and in the weeks that followed we learned a lot of things on dieting down through the centuries.

ELMER DELVES DEEPER

Remember how I caught myself pulling a lot of fat boy's tricks back there aways?

How I caught myself trying to walk erect so as to look taller and justify my heft? How I tried to look slimmer by trimming my hair instead of my lard? How I window-shopped for shoes with built-up heels?

All fat boys' tricks.

Well, once I'd organized the F. B. I., I threw the entire resources into studying fat boy psychology.

Only by looking ourselves squarely in our pouchy eyes and calling the turn on all the dodges we used to conceal and ignore and minimize our bay-windows, bulges, and spare tires could we force ourselves to face facts and stop thinking like fatheads.

FAT BOYS ARE SENSITIVE

There are three classifications of fat folks:

Bewildered—he wonders how he got that way.
Embarrassed—the fellow who tries to hide his lard.
Face Saver—says it runs in the family.

Little Known Facts on Fat Boys

Now fat boys don't mind being called "fat boys"—but don't call them "fat men."

Few even admit to being fat. They call it "muscles."

They hate to have you constantly want them to go on a diet. Ever know a drunkard who liked to be around people who kept saying, "Don't you know demon rum is ruining you?"

And, like drunkards, fat boys with caloric jags on day after day will not take a Calorie Cure until they make up their minds they want to.

You can't force 'em to diet. They detest the word. But once they toss down their knife and fork some night with a, "*I have made up my mind to get thin,*" then they can be saved. Only then will they take on our F. B. I. motto: "Eat tomorrow!"

"INSIDE ELMER"

Maybe I'm ripe for a book, *Inside Elmer*—or better yet, *Inside Fat Boy*.

Perhaps *Fat Boy Confidential* might be good, too, for my next book, only there is nothing confidential about a fat hind end.

Losing weight is "big business"—and I mean big!

For a guest and a calorie are most noticeable on the third day.

It takes 36 hours, you know, for food you eat today to walk and talk inside fat boys, as I've told you before.

What are some other interesting and little-known

Little Known Facts on Fat Boys

facts that might help Big Blimps keep off weight by giving them more knowledge?

Did You Know?

Since the days of Rome, dieting fads have come and gone with great regularity.

In England they had "groaning tables" where you sat, and when you ate too much and got a tummy ache you were in the right spot to groan.

In Grandmaw's time there came the lamb-chop fad, then pineapple, then boiled eggs, the Hollywood diet, and even Paul Whiteman's soup diet.

Along came the mechanical age and its rolling-pin methods of shifting weight, plus thumpers and bumpers, and now pills and rubber blankets.

Are these fads and methods any good? I'll leave this up to you.

I just recall old Walt Whitman's remark (he was a doctor, too, as well as a poet), when he told a patient always self-administering for his ailments from health articles: "Watch out you don't die from a *misprint!*"

Amazing But True!

That divorced people often put on great weight. It seems after an emotional crisis such as death, divorce, a shock, illness, you overeat.

Many a fallen fat boy might look into his "emotions"

Little Known Facts on Fat Boys

for the reason he dieted successfully, only to gain it back.

So when you see one drowning his soul in a mess of hamburgers, ask him is he still married?

"Families" are often the cause of overweight. You visit your relatives, and if you don't eat you are an outcast.

There is truth to the song: "If I Knew You Were Coming I'd 'a' Baked a Cake"!

Fat Boy Advice: *Don't tell 'em when you are coming!*

Other Fat Makers!

The present-day automobiles, dish and clothes washers, and fancy ironers, put on weight.

You have to expend less calories today in the kitchen.

Of course, few fat boys are ever found in the kitchen other than near another Twentieth Century wonder, the refrigerator.

Even airplane pilots can "set the ship" and wander back by the stewardess for a few calories!

And they even have coaster brakes now on bicycles, so teenager doesn't have to pump so much and can take the moment to down a hot dawg!

The fireman on a Diesel engine has far less calories to expend than his predecessor on the old Iron Horse with shovel and coal.

Watch out, fat folks, only a Turk likes 'em chubby!

Little Known Facts on Fat Boys

Causes of the Burp!

The fat boy's "give away" is the burp, outspoken or hidden behind a joke.

What causes them? That is, what kinds of food?

Our F. B. I. finds these are the burp-making foods:

        cabbage   cauliflower
        turnips   onions
        Brussels sprouts   melons

One fatso has found that foods that give off strong odors as they are being cooked, emitting gas, are good burp-makers.

Come to think of it, you can smell cabbage a block away, onions three blocks, turnips four blocks and sprouts all the way back to Brussels.

But these same items eaten raw don't seem, according to docs, to contain as much gas as when brewed.

No wonder no one burped in *Tobacco Road!*

FATSO'S GAIN IS HIS LOSS

One reason fatso regained his weight is because of the false criticism of his friends—his fat ones—as I've indicated all along.

It is hard to stand a siege of such remarks as:

    You used to look important—like an executive.
    You look run-down—been sick lately?
    You look wan and worried—lose money?

Little Known Facts on Fat Boys

Fatso must learn to overcome the jealousies of his fat friends who have lacked his courage.

For his gain is usually his loss! Which is why he should quit hobnobbing with his fat friends, just as an alcoholic should stop hanging around with his drinking cronies.

When a fat friend holds up a piece of apple pie and says, "Don't you wish you could eat it?" that is real temptation for an old fatso.

Which is why we organized our Fallen Fat Boys' Society.

Together we lose!

P. S. Have you joined yet?

BEING A CALORIE THIEF ONLY BRINGS ON GRIEF—*Poor Elmer's Almanac.*

13

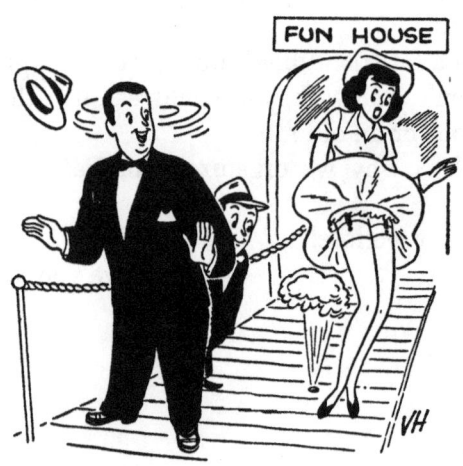

The Fat Boy's Gymnasium

I used to be a sales-booster instead of a diet-croaker.

People asked me to help them sell something—to find the sizzle in onions, rowboats, bunion pads, Mexican jumping beans—any drug on the market.

Now I'm "Doc Diet" to many.

The Fat Boy's Gymnasium

People now want to know how many calories in Camembert, a dried prune, or Swedish pancakes.

True, a salesman with a second suitcase is apt to bog down before he arrives in time to make a sizzling sale, only to find that Slim Jim, toting a midget-size briefcase, got the order.

But, in the main, the title of "diet editor" has replaced my title of "sales sizzler."

Where they used to write me, "How can I sell leftover Army goods?" now I get letters asking: "How can I tighten up my leftover chins?"

TRUE LOW-DOWN ON EXERCISE

Exercise is mainly for bull fighters, track men, tumblers, and burlesque "fall guys."

If exercise really takes off weight, why is Aunt Emmy sporting three chins? And the way she talks, too?

Why are wrestlers big fellows when they get more workouts per night than a Y. M. C. A. director?

This should settle once and for all the exercise question, especially when I retell you that:

> You must walk 36 miles . . .
> Bend over 25,000 times . . .
> Play 216 holes of golf . . .

To lose one little stinking pound of fat. You may sweat off five pounds of water, but that comes right on at the 19th hole—maybe even before.

The Fat Boy's Gymnasium

You must ride a horse 41 hours to lose the pound. Of course, if you're the horse you'll lose 10 or so!

Did you know if you are 40 pounds overweight, you can lose it by bending over 10 times after each meal—and in 75 years you will have lost the 40 pounds?

And when you swim the English Channel, you are only four pounds of FAT lighter.

REAL VALUE OF EXERCISE

But aside from toning up the system, making you feel like Atlas on the loose, or Bernarr MacFadden in the raw, exercise does have its value.

Exercise hardens fat—and makes you hungry.

But in so doing, it does tighten up the muscles and skin, and pulls in the flaps under your chin and where the spare tire left a few rolls of flesh.

So for the fallen fat boy—spare on fat now—but lousy with wrinkles, here are some exercises:

THE FAT-BOY EXERCISES

1. Triple-Chin Exercise:

This is a weak—and obvious spot—on the anatomy of a fat boy, his chubby mate, or tubby teenager. Merely opening and closing the mouth has little effect.

So try this. Push the chin way out; pull it back. Then circle the head right, then left. This is guaranteed, if done several times a day, to get you down to your last chin.

The Fat Boy's Gymnasium

But remember the fat won't leave the body. It just shifts to another spot.

That spot? Well, it's apt to be the hips.

2. *Elmer's Hip Hula:*

Put the hands behind your head. Then roll the entire body around in circles, first left, then right.

Soon the hips will tighten up. You'll be down a size or two in clothing.

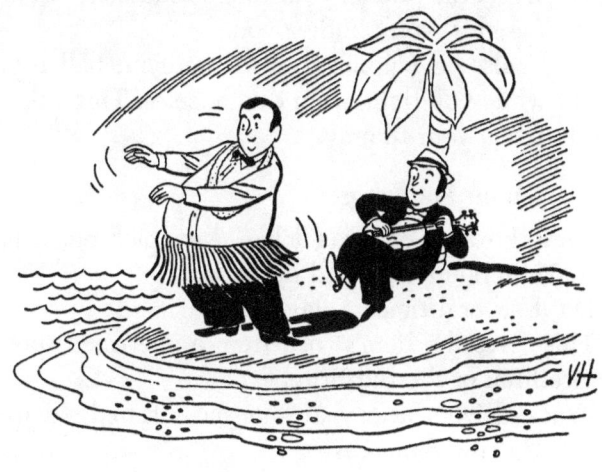

Remember Little Egypt, boys?

3. *Elmer's Tummy Bumps:*

Now the Hip Hula won't cause fat to melt off the hips. It just shifts it to another fat-boy weak spot . . . the tummy!

The Fat Boy's Gymnasium

So push the tummy out; then back. Many times. In elevators to get more space. While driving the car. You gotta do something then anyway.

Soon the bay window will disappear. Never saw one on a burlesque bumper, did you?

Here's another one: Lie in bed, raise the legs together. Now let them down, but not quite to the bed. Repeat several times.

You'll feel the pull on your tummy muscles, but after a few days this won't bother you.

Might also have junior throw a medicine ball at your midriff while you tighten up the muscles. This will also help toughen your tummy.

4. The Fanny Fandango:

Here, boys, is one you'll like. You pick out a hard chair. Then bounce up and down on it.

Do it several times a day.

This gives the bum's rush from a cherished spot on the Brethren of the Big Britches.

Truck drivers nearly always have lean hind quarters. So do cow punchers.

They're constantly bouncing up and down. Nothing to stop a 200-pound fatso from doing the same thing!

P. S.—Should you open a door suddenly and see the fat boss battering his seat on a chair, don't yell for the paddy wagon or a brace of Dr. Kildare's.

He's perhaps warding off that secretary's spread!

The Fat Boy's Gymnasium

TIGHTENING UP THE OTHER LOOSE SKIN

Skin hanging on the thighs, the arms—wherever your fat has left you—can be removed by simple exercises.

Example: Push the arms out in front of you. Pull them back. Now stretch them out sideways and level with your shoulders. Move them around in circles. Repeat 20 times or so.

Then you might wash out a few sets of long underwear using an old-fashioned scrub board!

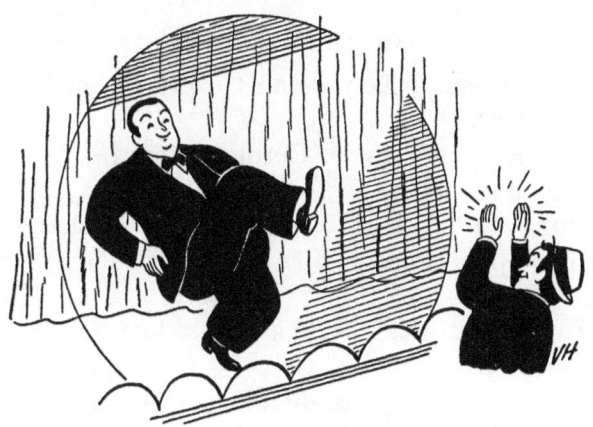

Take a 10-minute break. On second thought, you'll probably need a month's vacation in Florida!

If your arthritis permits, squat a few times a day—like Jack in the Box. This'll tighten up leg flab.

The Fat Boy's Gymnasium

Don't forget to come back up! People look odd walking around in a squat position.

Then stand on one leg and circle the other leg. Kick like a chorus girl.

Remember to put the other leg down when you reverse the procedure!

Any exercise that moves the muscles under flabby skin is bound to be beneficial. Soon your wrinkles will be ironed out.

You'll be as smooth as you were the day the doc slapped you and announced: "It's a boy!"

HAIL THE HAMMOCK!

Keep in mind: Exercise ain't worth a hoot for lopping off lard.

Calories put it there. Cutting calories is the only way to take it off.

Sure, you "work off" some suet. But I mean work!

If you play handball from five to seven hours, you'll lose a pound.

You have to roller skate a mile to lose the effect of one hot roll!

Our F. B. I. reports there are 4,000 calories to a pound. So, if you are 20 pounds overweight you have a "coal bin" of 80,000 excess calories to "burn off."

You can do this by walking 720 miles—without eating!

You have to walk 36 miles to lose a single pound.

The Fat Boy's Gymnasium

That's as far as from Dallas to Fort Worth. And who would go to Fort Worth—even if it meant losing 10 pounds! *

Fort Worth, incidentally, is the home of the Fat Boy Range Hand.

He's the chubby cowboy who uses a six-shooter belt to hold up his pot. He sticks his thumbs in his belt, proudly pushes out his paunch and says: "Howdah, Podnah!"

Fat boys in Dallas occasionally lose an ounce or so chasing after a blonde in front of Neiman-Marcus. In Fort Worth, steer roping continues to be the main sport.

Anyway, we fallen fat boys of the F. B. I. still hail The Hammock. In it we banish all thoughts of undue exercise—and scheme out ways to cut down on calories.

"FAT AND FORTY"

This means that after 40 you don't *mind* watching the effects of wind machines in the Fun House, or the show gals at the grocerymen's annual smoker.

But you wouldn't crane your neck to see the scenery. Your movements slow down. You burn less calories. But you still eat like the Romeo you were!

Eat less, you'll live longer and see more sights in life.

Your eyes will follow the whoosh and swirl of the wind down Main Street on blustery days.

* In case you haven't heard, Dallas and Fort Worth, Texas' "twin" cities, are always fussin' and feudin'. Elmer lives in Dallas.

The Fat Boy's Gymnasium

YOU'LL LOOK YEARS YOUNGER

Fat men not only *act* older than their years: they *look* older.

Consider those perennial juveniles of the movies. Jack Haley, for example. The guy must be 200 years old, yet his trim physique makes him look young.

When Fattie Arbuckle died, he was a young man. But he didn't *look* young.

People used to criticize my wife for "letting your pore 'ol pappy mow the lawn!"

That was *me* they were talking about. Elmer, the Beanery Blimp.

Since I switched from fat to slim and became a Beau Brummell about town, folks think my spouse switched hubbies.

It's fun being taken for your kid brother again!

And acting like him!

Insurance people will tell you that you grew 10 years younger when you slid down the weight scale.

Tarn me loose, I see a redhead!

IF AND WHEN YOU NO LONGER SAG,
THEN SURE AS HECK YOU'VE A RIGHT TO BRAG.
—*Poor Elmer's Almanac* (contributed by his secretary).

14

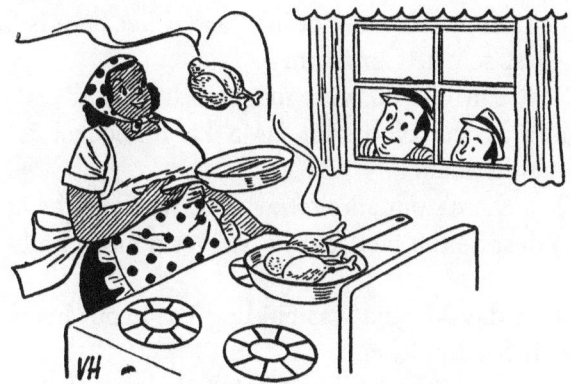

Don't Shoot the Cook— She's Your Best Friend

Jack Benny has his Rochester.

I have Martha, our 300-pound cook, to provide comic relief and an occasional calorie quip.

She's particularly unmanageable after a session listening to Beulah on the radio.

And we of the Dallas Chapter of the F. B. I. have about given up trying to convert her.

Don't Shoot the Cook—She's Your Best Friend

Not long ago, she observed:

"When you is young you eats and wonders where it is all goin'. But when you gets older, you realizes it went all over you."

She's often said she doesn't care if her man is fat or thin—"jest so's he's breathin'."

What can you do with someone like that?

She's as shy of dieting as a knob-knocker is of a plain-clothesman.

Then there's our stable-boy, Pat, who weighs in wet at 145 despite the fact that he swings a mean knife and fork.

Other day Martha was chiding Pat about his eating so much fried chicken.

"You knows the hens can hatch the eggs that makes them little fryers faster'n you can eat 'em," she said. "You can't hope to eat 'em all!"

Pat raised his head from the plate just long enough to grunt:

"Nope. But I shore has them hens worried. They is workin' nights now!"

That's calorie life at Sizzle Ranch.

MARTHA'S TOO BIG TO HIDE

Martha detracts about half a ton from my prestige every time she stands out by the highway waiting for the bus.

Don't Shoot the Cook—She's Your Best Friend

But our local F. B. I. chapter wouldn't exchange her for any other mascot.

She's too much fun!

Recently one of my reforming fat boy friends caught Martha flirting with a neighbor's yardman.

"Martha," my friend warned, "remember that men are no good. They are just two-legged animals."

When she had recovered from a prolonged fit of laughter, Martha replied:

"Yassuh. But they shore makes fine house pets!"

She listens to Beulah too much!

I don't know whom Pat listens to, but the other day he was running up and down the yard hollering, "Hey! Hey!"

We all went out to see what was up. The barn was on fire.

"You silly boy!" said Martha, "why didn't you holler fire?"

"I couldn't think of the word!" Pat says.

Oh, well. We couldn't have saved the barn anyway.

MARTHA OFTEN READS THE "DIET ACT"

While Martha would consider it snobbery to pass up a pork chop, she doesn't mind what other people do. I'll say that much for her.

And she's on my side, even tho it's the "suicide." Just so I don't try to ration her vittles.

She often amuses herself by reading the reducing

Don't Shoot the Cook—She's Your Best Friend

rules to my fatso friends, using herself as a ghastly example of what could happen to them.

"That you kin have ten bowls of this thin chicken soup to one of that creamed-up stuff?"

"That you kin have eight helpings of caviar to one fried poke chop, but who wants to help them Russians anyhow?"

Then as she passes me on her way to the kitchen she'll lean close and whisper:

"How'm ah doin', Boss?"

Even Martha knows that the "pot likker" off vegetables is too valuable in vitamins to throw away. So she bastes it on the vegetables just as she serves them.

Which is why I said, don't shoot the cook!

She's your best friend even if she is your wife!

GETTING FAT IS A "DISEASE"

That's Martha's way of explaining why she is fat.

"All us chubby folks has our alibis—and that's mine," she says, laughing. "I'm just unallergic to food!"

Martha is dead right. Desire for food is the downfall of fat boys.

But for our family she broils—realizing that the grease drips into the flames instead of onto our plates—and boils.

She crisps our bacon so that it drops from a possible 75 calories per slice to just 25.

Don't Shoot the Cook—She's Your Best Friend

"I keeps the boss man outa the fry pan," she says, "but fo the life of me ah can't keep myself out!"

Martha admits she likes to eat "high on the hog." That's where the fat is!

A GOOD COOK CAN HELP YOU

It's just like getting the doctor on your side when you are sick—or the judge when you are pinched for speeding.

She went downtown "trading" one day, and returned with an assortment of pots and pans designed to drain off fat in the cooking process.

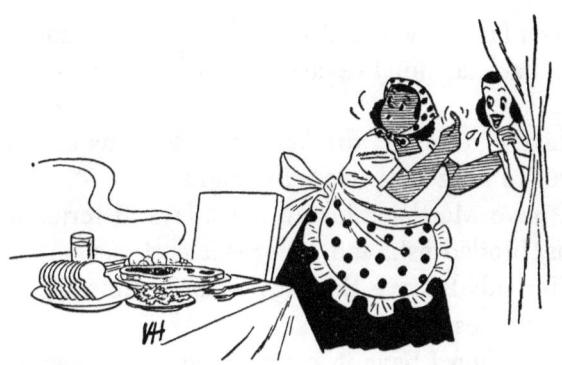

Better look into this. There are many utensils that do away with the calorie before it can hit the table. While I was waging that first grim Battle of the

Don't Shoot the Cook—She's Your Best Friend

Bulge, my slender wife, Beth, used to yearn for foods that were forbidden on our menu.

She'd sneak into the kitchen for an occasionally steak smothered in butter, or a piece of apple strudel smothered in lard sauce. Martha would console her.

"Don't get sore at him," she'd say. "Eatin' is his passion—jus' lak kissin' is a passion to others."

Then Martha would get starry-eyed.

"Today's poke chop is tomorrow's fat—same as kissin' tonight in the moonlight is tomorrow's weddin' ring!"

MARTHA IS MY DIET DICTATOR

As a fat boy who lost his bulges, relaxed, and gained them back again, I've learned to lean heavily on the cook.

Like a reformed drinker often depends on the bartender to keep him steered straight.

I have Martha thinking nowadays in terms of thin soups, broiled fish, and lean meat portions.

Her salads have thin, low-calorie dressings instead of thick ones.

Pie, when I have it, comes from the kitchen in gentleman-size slices.

She can take some low-caloried raw materials that might have tasted like a dried-up mop, and fix them so they're almost as savory as chicken pot pie.

Don't Shoot the Cook—She's Your Best Friend

Her fatless stews, made of lean meat, spices and fresh vegetables, are out of this world!

After we let the caloric traces down the other night by way of celebrating my near-victory over fat, I heard Martha singing in the kitchen:

> Everything's rosy and sweet again,
> 'Cause the boss man's weight is normal,
> And he's on his feet again!

So keep on the good side of whoever is custodian of your pots and pans—otherwise, like Lucrezia Borgia, they might slip you a fast caloric Mickey Finn.

Martha makes us all laugh off several pounds a year.

During her vacation trip to New York she refused to ride on the top of the Fifth Avenue Bus.

"Not for this fat gal," she said. "There ain't no driver up there!"

"I GOT GLANDS!"

Another typical Martha alibi:

"It isn't that wheelbarrow load of food fat folks eat every day! It's their glands."

F.B.I. research indicates it isn't weak-working glands that produce fat, so much as over-worked glands that cripple their proper functioning.

Fat-sabotaged glands maladjust your metabolism. Your "motor" stops running efficiently, fails to burn up all the calories you pour into your "carburetor."

Don't Shoot the Cook—She's Your Best Friend

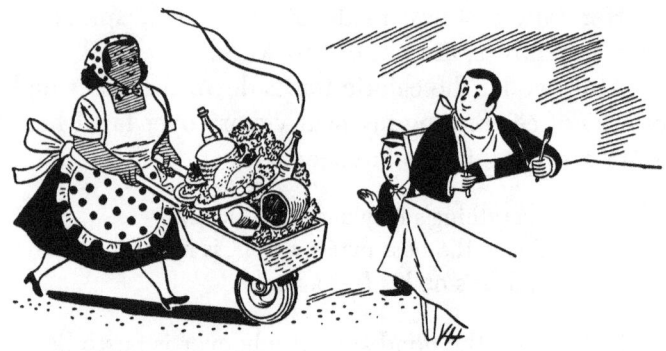

May as well face the facts, fat folks!

Unburned calories may be likened to carbon in a cylinder. They pile up in the form of fat.

MARTHA'S CLAN GATHERS AROUND

Now Martha is kinda king pin in the neighborhood, living with the man who wrote *The Fat Boy's Book*.

Her cronies gather up here, especially a few fat ones. There's Mary down the street. Three hundred pounds of bad local testimonial for me.

But Julie—well, all wet she isn't over 120. Bill, her daughter, turns in a neat figure, but she realizes she is in bad company with Mary and her calories on one side of her, and Martha and hers on the other side.

As will happen, they prime me with questions, the latest of which is, "How about them thyroid tablets? Do they really take off weight?"

Well, here's the real low-down.

Don't Shoot the Cook—She's Your Best Friend

THYROID IS LIKE A THERMOSTAT

I'm not a doc. I can only tell you what he tells me.

Which in simple cook's language is that your thyroid, located in your neck, is like a "thermostat."

If there's lots of thyroid secretion, your motor runs at high speed and you burn up calories faster.

The thyroid, you see, governs your speed of living.

If thyroid is lacking, your motor idles—you walk slower, stand up less, and thus burn up fewer calories.

Now don't run for the iodine bottle!

Don't be a medicine-chest experimenter, a self-made guinea pig.

See your doc.

Maybe if thyroid is your trouble, the doc can help your thermostat back to perfect running order.

He might recommend iodized salt, sea foods, Vitamin A or B, or thyroid tablets themselves.

But don't count on this being your trouble. It's perhaps 40 pounds of dead-weight that is slowing you up.

A "second suitcase"!

WHEN FAT IS INEVITABLE RELAX AND ENJOY IT—*Poor Martha's Almanac.*

15

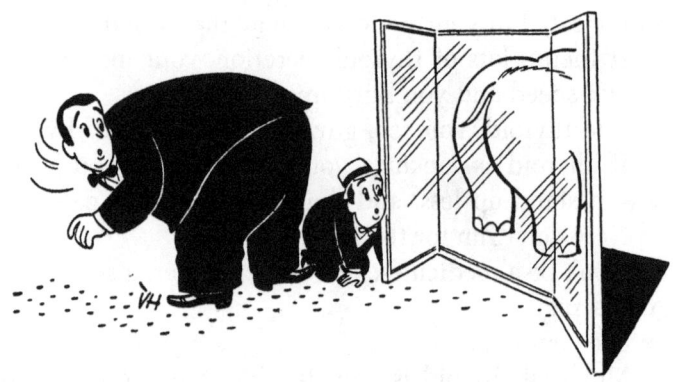

Fat Boys Can Eat Desserts

One Fat Boy Lament is more common than all the rest.

"I'd lose a ton if I didn't have a sweet tooth!"

This is a futile cry from our pudgy populace.

The yen for sweets, like sex and the Straits of Gibraltar, seems here to stay.

Yet, all is not lost for us fat-saddled citizens!

Don't pass up that mint parfait before you hear me out!

Fat Boys Can Eat Desserts

We fallen fat boys of the F.B.I., addicted to dessert delights, put our pineapple upside-down cakes at parade rest and set out to learn some sugary, fat-foiling facts.

We discovered that you *can* have your cake and eat it too!

BUT . . .

. . . we fatsos gotta handle desserts with extra care.

No blind wading through a mire of banana splits, crepe suzettes and creamy pastry concoctions.

Unless we want another compartment added to our steamer trunk derrières!

There's cunning involved in getting chummy with desserts.

There are tummy-trimming tricks of the trade.

And the greatest gimmick of them all is KNOWING the caloric content of your favorite desserts.

HOW TO EAT DESSERTS

Edit your sweet-tooth satisfiers.

Know their caloric tariff!

Then fit them into your booster diet scheme along with all other foods.

For example, you're drowning your eye teeth drooling for a certain 300-calorie dessert.

You just gotta have it!

Okay. Lap it up, and may the marshmallow whip drip where it may.

Fat Boys Can Eat Desserts

But then be a good sport.

"Pay" for it by deducting the 300 calories from your daily diet allowance.

Then your body won't send you a "bill" in the form of a retread on your spare tire!

If you skim calories all along the line of your daily munching, you can eat a calorie-packed dessert and be none the worse for wear.

A 100-calorie hunk of Camembert, a 150-calorie scoop of vanilla ice cream or a 500-calorie socko of mince pie are fine and dandy.

But don't think you can eat them "on the cuff." Fat boys have no calorie credit!

And naturally, if you do like my Grandpa Strobel and eat pie three times a day, be sure you're chopping down trees in between meals to burn up some of the calories.

Once a day on desserts is okay for us fat boys—because we know their fat-forming ratios.

We tote up the calories, be they many or few.

And in each case, we subtract—so that we don't add weight.

SLICE OFF THE FROSTING

Now we get into some of the finer points of foiling a dessert calorie.

One nifty trick: Slice the frosting off cake—just like you trim the fat off a ham steak.

Fat Boys Can Eat Desserts

Give the frosting to Junior. He needs it for energy to get into mischief.

Eat fruit with a fork, and don't sop up the sweet juices.

If you have a choice between pound cake and chocolate—take the pound, and save ounces.

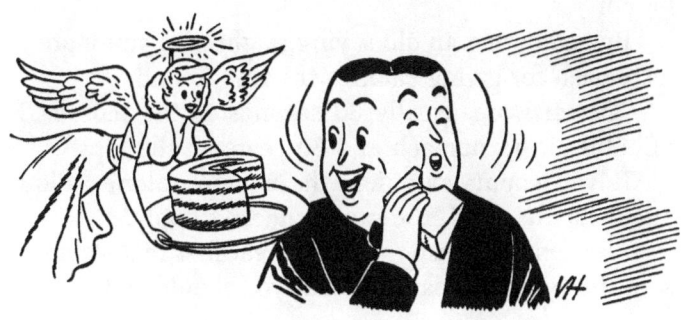

Angel food cake is friendly to fat boys. Like pound cake, it's spare in calories.

But slice the icing!

As I mentioned in our Bible (*The Fat Boy's Book*), the best way to judge a hunk of pie at a glance is to give it about 100 calories per inch of crust around the outer edge.

Custard pies are a little less; pecans and minces somewhat more per inch.

Restaurant servings of cheese are usually around 100

calories, the creamed ones like Camembert more, solid varieties, like American, somewhat less.

That grated cheese you dump on onion soup or spaghetti ranges around 100 per spoonful—so just because you aren't measuring it exactly, don't think it isn't going to make your measurements bigger!

You can't kid a calorie! (Calories have no sense of humor.)

Remembering an old saying might give you more of a stomach for giving calories the run-around:

"Desserts are usually 30 seconds in the mouth, 30 minutes in the stomach and 30 years on the hips."

If you count your desserts in your calorie "allowance" for the meal, the saying doesn't apply.

(Remember, it isn't what you eat first that stacks on suet! It's what you eat last—that you shouldn't.)

DESSERTS WHILE ON A DIET?

Certainly. If you will only tally them up on The Fat Boy's Thermometer.

Obviously, however, you'll be better off cutting your desserts in half during your booster battle.

A little sweet stuff goes a long way. (All around your 38th parallel.)

Sweets satisfy the inner man—make the meal feel complete.

In fact, the docs tell me a little sweets will slow up your digestion. This means food stays longer in the

Fat Boys Can Eat Desserts

tummy and keeps you from getting hungry quite so soon.

I ate a dab of sweets while losing my 40 pounds in 80 days, and always left the table feeling "satisfied."

Eating desserts is like wearing sun glasses. You "double-cross" nature a little and feel better for having done it.

CHEESE IT! THE CALORIES!

Cheese eating has thwarted many a well-intentioned fat boy.

The hazard is identical with the one encountered during the social drinking hour.

It's not so much what the right hand is doing, but what the left is undoing!

Cocktail in the right hand, the left hand unconsciously grubs around for tidbits—which total up to a big calorie binge. A handful of bar nibbles can go as high as two highballs.

Cheese in the right hand, the left gropes for something to put it on, dab it with, or dip it in.

Often the 100-calorie sliver of cheese in the right hand becomes just a "base" for a whole bunch of "unconscious" calories.

"Unconscious" calories suddenly come to life inside you!

We F.B.I. fellows prefer a slice of apple to rest our cheese on.

Fat Boys Can Eat Desserts

LOW CALORIED DESSERTS—THE FAT BOY'S PENANCE

No food lover is fond of those "hospital desserts."

You know, those fancy custards and imitation gelatines. They look too "tea-roomy" for a he-man's appetite.

On a strict diet, though, they do the job.

Better stick with them—pay your penalty for years of feasting.

Custards and certain gelatines are your penance—during the 21 lenten days of your booster diet.

Fruit makes a good dessert, too. It fills the sweet tooth.

Beware! Stay aloof from canned fruits laden with sugary syrups, unless you count them honestly and then eat within your calorie allowance.

Read the labels on grapefruit cans. A glass of grapefruit juice contains only 50 calories—but that means UNSWEETENED.

Fruits like prunes that have been dried, then cooked and sweetened, are heavy in calories.

Best way is to eat your fruit as it comes off the tree.

EMILY POST WON'T APPROVE

Just as you lose calories when you eat fruit from a fork, instead of a spoon, you lose calories when you choose crumb instead of chocolate cake.

Time you get finished wrestling with a good crumb cake, half of it is all over the table and the rest on old fatso's vest.

Fat Boys Can Eat Desserts

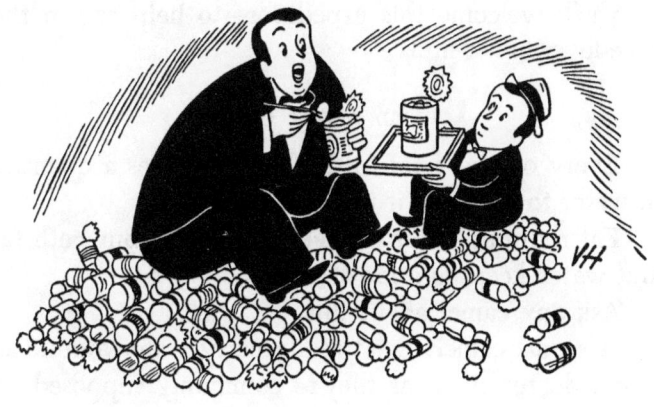

It took one of our F.B.I. agents to think up that trick!

The idea is all in keeping with the Fallen Fat Boy's chant:

> Less on the fork and more on the plate;
> That's the big secret of losing weight.

The agent undoubtedly got inspiration from another saying in *Poor Elmer's Almanac:*

> Take Elmer's advice:
> Shake your salads twice!

Get the lady in your kitchen to comb the grocery shelves for some of those delectable, low-caloried desserts during your Big Britches Battle.

Fat Boys Can Eat Desserts

She'll welcome this expedition—to help regain the lithe lover in her life!

A WORD ABOUT CAMELS

Every ounce of fat in the body requires a quantity of water to maintain it in the tissues.

Fat requires water to "keep in shape"—but both fat and water keep *you* out of shape.

Ask any camel about this.

It seems camels don't really carry water around in an inside reservoir, as they're commonly supposed to.

The water camels tap during a long desert trek is really fat in their humps. As they hump along over the sand dunes, the fat burns and turns to water.

It's the same with humans. Even though they don't have humps, when they lose fat they lose water weight.

Our F.B.I. had to visit a zoo to find this out!

Muscles, too, require water to keep fit. The bigger the muscle, the more water it causes to be retained in the tissues.

So you can see how weight-lifting—building a blacksmith's muscles—can't help you lose weight! (*I'm strictly a hammock athlete, myself!*)

Body tissues, the docs say, are "water storage tanks."

That candy bar you eat, over and above your daily calorie quota, often requires four times its own weight in water when it turns into fat and is stored up!

Fat Boys Can Eat Desserts

And any fat boy knows a pint is a pound the world around.

Even the bones in your body are 40 per cent water!

Our F.B.I. is now trying to find out how much water is in that skeleton in Grandma's closet!

P.S.—I'm nearing 186 again!

GET UP FROM THE TABLE,
LEAVE IT FLAT!
THAT'S THE BOSS MAN'S SECRET
FOR REMOVING FAT.

—*Poor Martha's Almanac.*

16

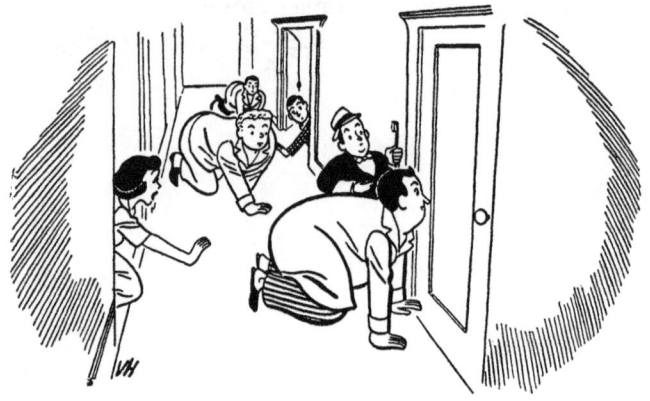

Elmer Answers His Mailbag

I got fat.

I had given the world the low-down on how to diet. Then, seemingly, I gained back what others lost.

People, noticing my protruding paunch, branded me a charlatan—a fatty fraud.

My only consolation for a time was letters—mailbags full of them coming to my desk from other fallen fat boys.

Elmer Answers His Mailbag

In a short time more than 3,000,000 letters arrived from the 200 newspapers that serialized the diet story.*

I couldn't begin to answer every one. But when I found a similarity in questions, I mimeographed the answers and sent them out.

Here are a few typical queries and the substance of my replies:

QUESTION: Will hot breads fatten you faster than cold ones?

ANSWER: Hot or cold, they have the same calorie count.

QUESTION: Will smoking cause you to lose weight?

ANSWER: Smoking gives your metabolism a slight lift, which tends to keep you "on the go." Motion burns up calories.

QUESTION: Will food you eat late at night fatten you faster?

ANSWER: It isn't what time you eat—but how much.

QUESTION: Will sleeping after eating add weight faster?

ANSWER: No—but rest helps digestion.

QUESTION: Will water before or during meals help make you fat?

* Editor and Publisher claimed this broke an all-time record in the history of journalism.

Elmer Answers His Mailbag

ANSWER: There are no calories in sunshine or tap water. Water merely helps fill up the tummy. Each glass weighs one-half pound, but the weight is only temporary.

QUESTION: Can you mix proteins with carbohydrates?

ANSWER: You sure can—and pickles with ice cream!

QUESTION: Do babies make women fat?

ANSWER: New findings indicate expectants should not gain more than about 16 pounds.

QUESTION: What is the difference in lard you buy and the lard that is on you?

ANSWER: Probably about $10 a pound. The lard you buy costs maybe 21¢. Lard you "manufacture" costs a heck of a lot more. The fat boy who pats his tummy and says, "This cost me $20,000," may not be kidding.

"YA GOTTA HAVE A HOT MEAL"

Perhaps the greatest number of kicks and hollers come to me from fat boys who claim they just "gotta have a hot meal."

Nonsense!

Sometimes the Army goes for days with cold rations.

Elmer Answers His Mailbag

Seldom do I serve hot foods to the dog—yet he never burps!

Sorry, fat boys, it just isn't so.

Another big question is, "Will five meals—small ones—per day thin a fellow faster than a big one?"

The answer: It isn't the frequency with which you guzzle calories that puts on weight. It's how many and how often.

Of course, one big meal dumped suddenly into the stomach is apt to cause the burps faster than if you ate the equivalent amount of food at intervals.

THE WORLD'S GREATEST LOVE

It's the love of one fat boy for another.

The sympathy, the attention each gives the other, is almost as classical as the affair of Damon and Pythias, Antony and Cleopatra or Sid Caesar and Imogene Coca!

There is a real fusing of souls when two sad-faced fat boys get together to discuss the latest diet fads—and swap the newest burp pills.

So when a fellow fat boy bares his soul—or breadbasket—and asks such questions as the following, he deserves an honest answer:

QUESTION: How can I break the icebox habit?
ANSWER: Put a padlock on it and give the key to the wife.
QUESTION: How can I stop burning candles at both ends?

Elmer Answers His Mailbag

ANSWER: Tie your hands behind your back and let your wife feed you as much as she thinks is good for you.

QUESTION: Is it true that the fatter you are the more you lose?

ANSWER: Sure—you have more excess suet to get off.

QUESTION: How can I break the habit of carrying sweets in my pocket?

ANSWER: Have your wife sew up the pocket!

LETTERS FROM FAT BOYS' WIVES

Some of the best letters that came my way after publication of *The Fat Boy's Book* were from wives.

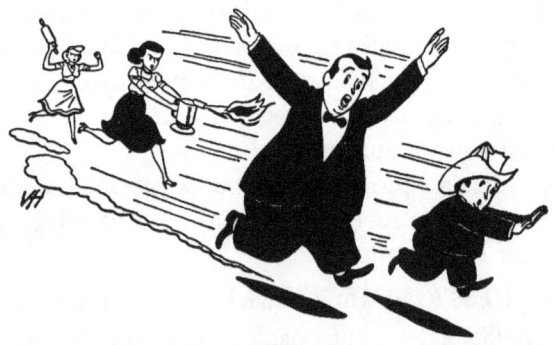

They scorched me for upsetting their cooking habits.

Assailed me for putting hubby up to his boyish tricks again.

Elmer Answers His Mailbag

Asked me for advice, since I had gotten their John into a diet dither.

For example:

QUESTION: How can I keep my Wilbur from the fourth helping? The fifth and sixth?

ANSWER: Cook just one helping. Or, if he won't stand for it, make him go to the kitchen for more. Most fat boys are too lazy to budge from the table.

QUESTION: How can I get Adelbert to talk more and eat less?

ANSWER: Every time he starts to shove something into his puss, ask him a question. Suggested: "How much is two and where can I get them?" "Are all your folks sloppy fat, too?"

QUESTION: My Lard Face refuses to exercise. What can I do?

ANSWER: Nothing. It'll only work up an appetite. As he thins down the urge to move around in yard or bedroom will return automatically.

QUESTION: How can I keep Bertram awake nights?

ANSWER: Don't change the subject, lady. I know your type! However, you might buy a Faye Emerson—or invite some widow over.

Elmer Answers His Mailbag

One letter sounds like a testimonial:

> Dear Elmer:
> Before Fulbright began using your dope, he never stayed awake three minutes at a stretch.
> Since he read your Fat Boy's fable, *I* haven't slept a wink.
> What do you suggest?

Boys will be boys. Especially reformed fat boys.

SOUR GRIPES

When you get a few million letters (*Elmer's book broke all records for reader response in newspaper history!*), you're bound to hear a sour note on and off.

Here's what I mean:

> Dear Judas Fat Boy:
> You're nuts! A menace to happy home life.
> My Jeremiah was a good boy until he read all the troubles he'd have if he kept his 300 pounds.
> So he reduced. Now I have all the troubles! He ain't home nights no more!
> Got an answer for that, Fat Boy's Home Wrecker?

Well, you can't please everybody. Sure as shootin', that pre-honeymoon look will come back into the old man's eyes in direct ratio to the fat that left his hide.

YOU CAN COAST—IF IT'S A ROAST—*Poor Elmer's Almanac.*

17

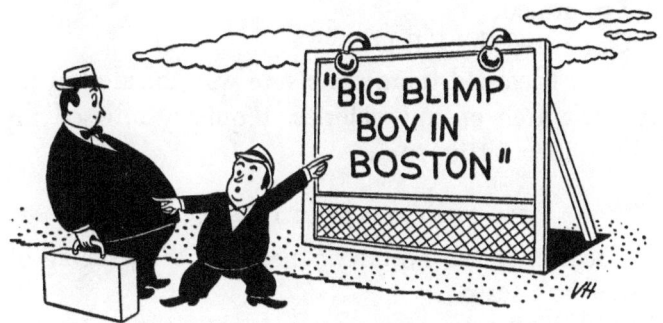

The Fat Boy's Kitchen

I had become King Size from eating small meals—the wrong kind.

"Big oaks from little acorns grow."

Same with big fat boys.

My width reflected the "broader" aspects of America's prosperity, you might say.

For a while there I was high man on the suet pole!

I lived a gay life, but you could hardly call me a "gay blade" any more.

I was more of a "solid citizen." Solid fat!

When I arrived in Boston for a speaking engage-

The Fat Boy's Kitchen

ment, my billing usually was "BIG BLIMP BOY IN BOSTON."

Then I hit the sawdust trail—the road back to fitness. I reformed.

Organized the F.B.I.

Soon I learned there's one sure way to sidestep the fat boy's arch enemy—calories. I quickly advised my fellow fallen fatties to . . .

KILL THE CALORIE IN THE KITCHEN

"Dead men tell no tales," the Injun said, slicing off the settler's scalp.

And dead calories carry no weight.

So we fat boys prevent our wives from unintentionally slipping us caloric shorts-stretchers by beating the calorie to the punch.

We invade the kitchen, watch food being made.

We put our vittles under the keenest of fat boys' observations.

The food squirms under our withering scrutiny!

Soon the hidden calories come out, hands up, ready to surrender.

Calories ain't so tough but what any fat boy can lick 'em!

SOME CALORIE-CATCHING TIPS

One of the best ways to frustrate a calorie is to strain it off the food, and down the kitchen drain.

The Fat Boy's Kitchen

Let it float out to sea and find some other victim!

Broiling fatty meats, like pork chops, enables us to sabotage calories—since much of the fat drips into the pan underneath.

Boiling meat also brings the calories out into the open—into the water. Then, before they can hide, we fat boys give them the bum's rush—into the sink.

Better down the kitchen pipes than down our pipes!

Practice Elmer's 3 B Method—Boil, Broil or Bake!

CHOICE OF INGREDIENTS IMPORTANT

A dish has only as many calories as the cook puts into it.

Therefore, we fat boys like to use up to one-fourth of soya flour with our wheat flour. Soya is low in calories.

And soya crackers have fewer calories than soda crackers.

The low-calorie breads are white, rye, and whole wheat.

French and Vienna loaves have still less.

It's biscuits, muffins, and corn bread that pack the powerful calorie punch!

Melba toast and Ry-Krisps have only 20 calories each. Guess Madame Melba had her operatic diet problems, too.

Gluten bread is the fat boy's friend—it has one-third less calories than other breads.

The Fat Boy's Kitchen

PICK LOW-CALORIE FOODS TO START WITH

Be choosey about what you eat!
This is perhaps the greatest diet secret of them all.

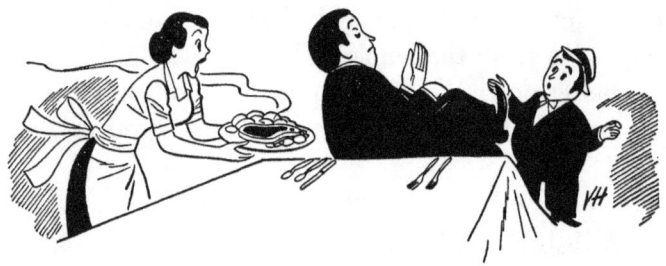

Know, for example, that Irish potatoes have fewer calories than sweet potatoes.

Maybe that's why the Irish are so full of blarney—they aren't too bogged down by calories to be lighthearted.

Mayonnaise is a high-calorie concoction—much higher than other salad dressings. Here is another place to fend off a calorie or two until the battle is over and you can lick up mayonnaise again like regular folks.

Dressings made with mineral oil and eggs have only four calories per tablespoon, compared with 75 to 100 for Roquefort dressings.

But my doc says, "Beware of mineral oil. It robs you of vitamin A by letting it slide away unabsorbed."

The Fat Boy's Kitchen

Our F.B.I. unearthed an interesting dietary fact: The foods that reduce most are the very foods highest in vitamins and minerals.

Meat, eggs, milk, cheese, green vegetables, cabbage, fruits.

Sauerkraut is good for fat boys. It's way low in calories—but like hay to a horse, it sure fills you up!

These are real ways to "catch the calorie in the act."

FOODS CAN FOOL YOU

You wouldn't drink water from a stream apt to carry the typhoid germ.

That's medical knowledge put to good use.

Similarly, we fat boys put our calorie knowledge to work for us.

We know, for example, that a tablespoonful of catsup has the same number of calories (25) as one ripe tomato, one-fourth cup of canned tomatoes or one-half cup of tomato juice.

That Liederkranz, Cheddar, Camembert and Pimento have fewer calories than Roquefort and Gruyère.

Being hep to calories this way keeps the little rascals from slipping slyly into our gizzards!

Perhaps the most interesting item our F.B.I. found on killing calories in the kitchen concerned meats.

Did you know that meat cooked rare has fewer calories than medium cooked meat? That medium steaks have fewer calories than well-done steaks?

The Fat Boy's Kitchen

The reason, it seems, is that by longer cooking the fat is "absorbed" into the meat. Fat on rare-cooked meat can easily be sliced away.

Another way to kill the calorie before it arrives at the table is to *omit* it.

Leave the icing off the cake, the chocolate syrup off the ice cream, the breading off the veal cutlets, the fat off the stew meat, etc.

You can also prepare food so that a calorie "goes further." For example, raw eggs run through the system so fast you hardly know you've eaten them.

So boil your eggs. They move slowest that way, and keep you feeling full longest.

A quick way to figure the calories in a hunk of meat is to allow 73 per ounce! That goes for nearly all meats.

Each ounce of meat, it seems, has, on the average, 28 calories of protein and 45 calories of fat.

Britain's inhabitants gained weight when their austerity program curtailed meat eating. Starches were substituted, and the results were often "tremendous!"

VIVE LA KNOWLEDGE

Fortified by calorie facts, we fat boys no longer enter into an eating session blindly.

We can "rap out" the pitfalls on a menu card quicker than a detective can spot a hot check chiseler.

We know now that the dark meat of chickens and

The Fat Boy's Kitchen

turkeys has more calories than the white—so we've become white-meat eaters.

Our F.B.I. also advises that:

Port and sherry have more calories per ounce than Scotch or bourbon, blended or bonded.

Even lettuce contains a calorie or two. The only kind that doesn't is that "long green" variety Uncle Sam takes away from you when you accumulate too much for your "health."

Nothing you eat—can take off weight!

Lobsters (with butter at a minimum) are good for fat boys. They're low in calories, and you burn some energy digging out the meat. But Newburg the old fellow, and you triple his calories!

Caviar doesn't add many calories (25 per teaspoonful), although it subtracts many pesos from your purse. The same quantity of other hors d'oeuvres "goop" might add 75 to 100 calories.

It pays to put the "grab" on pre-dinner celery and carrot tips. Your paw can hold only about 15 calories worth.

Stale bread has fewer calories than fresh—and because it crumbles easier, you gain by losing.

FAT BOY SCIENCE IS WONDERFUL

The docs have really gone all-out to help us hash-house hippos skin off our suet suits.

The Fat Boy's Kitchen

We're good for their business—and they're good for us.

A nice arrangement!

One dietitian found out that fat boys can take off their triple chins easier than fat gals can cut down on their corset circumference.

He didn't bother to find out how come!

Other slenderizing scientists found that nearly every fat boy has *one* weakness in his eating—just like some men have a weakness for blondes.

If each of us fatsos finds his own particular foible—maybe a fondness for malted milks or mid-meal munching—we can cut it out and start coming down.

Docs also have discovered that you have most difficulty reducing between the ages of 50 and 70.

Somehow the fat fellow in his fifties won't "stand still" for a tummy-trim as readily as his younger button-popping pals.

Guess those are the best-eating years of our lives! We usually have the money then, too—maybe that has something to do with it.

OTHER "DOC" DIET DISCOVERIES

That margarine and butter have the same number of vitamins, so take your choice, Podner!

Spinach has as much iron in it as Popeye says it does. But science has discovered that only a minute portion of all this iron can be utilized by the body.

The Fat Boy's Kitchen

"Hail the F.B.I.," say the nation's spinach-stuffed small fry.

Certain foods are inclined to make you burp, *viz.*, chocolates, onions, apples, cabbage, radishes (I love 'em), cucumbers, fats, greens such as collards and spinach. Even milk bothers some fat boys. They should be drinking buttermilk anyway!

However, docs say that often what is on your mind causes more indigestion and burps than what is on the fork!

So don't worry about next year's Christmas bills until the sheriff comes out to attach your golf clubs!

ELMER WHEELER DIET CONDITIONER

Here's a little three day diet to get you fat boys back on the Road to Success.

It is designed to shrink the stomach fast, yet keep you from wanting to gnaw off a desk leg.

It's very successful in our weight-control clinics around America.

Use for three days—or longer if you desire.

Breakfast:

Before breakfast each morning drink the juice of 1 lemon in a glass of hot water
4 Prunes—cooked without sugar—may use lemon
2 Eggs—poached or cooked (hard or soft) or scrambled over a double boiler, using no fat
1 Slice Toast, whole grain

The Fat Boy's Kitchen

1 Teaspoon Butter
Glass Skimmed Milk or Buttermilk (8 oz.)

Packed Lunch:
1 Hard Cooked Egg
Dill Pickles, Celery Sticks, and Carrot Sticks—all you want
6 Asparagus Spears—eat cold
1 Tomato
2 Pieces Melba Toast
Glass Skimmed Milk or Buttermilk (8 oz.)

4:00 P.M. Nibble Session:
1 Life Saver
1 Coke
Carrot and Celery Sticks

Dinner:
Glass Tomato Juice (8 oz.)
Broiled Lean Steak, or Hamburger Patty—well done and well drained—4 oz. raw weight
½ Cup Greens, Broccoli or Spinach
1 Cup Cabbage Slaw with Vinegar or Fat Boy's "Sweet-Sour Dressing"
Glass Skimmed Milk or Buttermilk (8 oz.)
1 Sliced Orange or ½ Grapefruit

Nite Nibble Session:
4 Prunes, as before
1 Life Saver

FAT IS NO LONGER FASHIONABLE

Years ago it was thought that the older you got the "bigger" you became—just naturally.

The Fat Boy's Kitchen

Now we know better—that the older we fatsos get the thinner we should become, so that our organs have less work to do.

It hasn't been so long since fat people were looked upon as prosperous people. A pot belly was a "sign of success."

Then the waltz was replaced by the mombo and rumba. The latter dances are hard on us fellers who are "out of shape."

The day of the 12-course meal faded as life became faster, and a big belly no longer makes the world regard us as the baron of all we survey.

Come to think of it, I guess we fat boys are just old-fashioned!

Can't you imagine one of us trying to get into one of those jet plane cockpits!

Guess we have to face it—we're still huffin' and puffin' along like freight trains in the jet-propelled age!

We of the F.B.I. have decided to adapt our torsos to the times. Why not join us?

Fat Boy Thermometer in hand, resolution in our hearts, let's get off it—and get on the booster diet.

What can we lose, except our fat?

IT'S BETTER TO HAVE FOUGHT FAT AND LOST, THAN NEVER TO HAVE BATTLED AT ALL. AT LEAST WE CAN SAY, "WE'RE VETERANS!"

DIETING: MIND OVER PLATTER—*Poor Elmer's Almanac.*

18

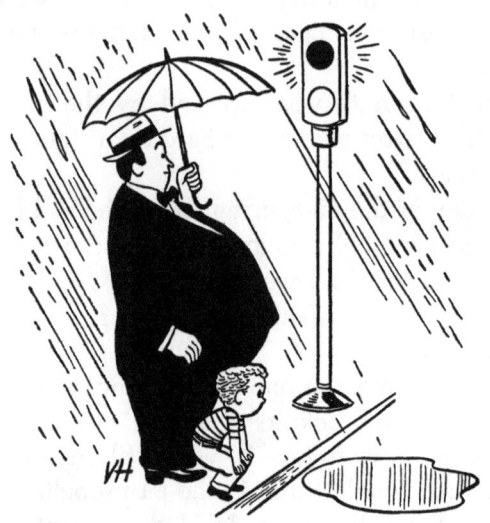

My Life with Girth

By Beth Wheeler

Editor's note: Women always get the last word, so we asked Mrs. Fat Boy to pass on her tips on how to handle chubby mates during their Battle of the Big Britches.

My Life with Girth

I had just begun writing a song titled "Rub-a-Dub-Dub, I Married a Tub," when that diet look came back on Elmer's face.

The song was to have been a sad ballad about life with a bay window.

What inspired it was that old triangle: (1) Elmer, (2) I, and (3) Elmer's indigestion.

One of us had to go. I recollected nothing in the marriage ceremony that obliged me to live with old Snooze Puss through "thick and thin," and then back to thick again.

Elmer's chances of impersonating a thin man were about 1,000 to 1. Kids used to stand under his balcony on rainy days waiting for street lights to change.

He almost had to use a cane to push doorbells.

Frankly, I began to feel I had married two men. I used to lie awake nights trying to remember how the other half lived.

By "other half" I mean the half of Elmer I originally married.

THAT "BETTER HALF" NONSENSE

I was getting sick and tired of being referred to as Elmer's "better half."

Better ONE THIRD would have been more accurate.

I learned firsthand that all blimps are not inflated with gas. Mine was solid suet.

My Life with Girth

Wedlock with a blimp *did* have its lighter moments, though. You'd have died laughing at Elmer calling for his dog for five minutes on end, when all the time the dog was right by his feet.

I must admit that sort of thing occasionally gave me a belly laugh, if you'll pardon the pun.

But certainly life with a fatso is no fiesta. It's more like a long-drawn-out siesta.

Old Eighth-of-a-Ton would chug home crammed to the ears with calories, light on the divan, and expire like a blown-out fuse.

Fat Boys are insomniacs in reverse.

Elmer never could keep awake long enough to chew the fat with friends of an evening. He just chewed the fat from his dinner plate, than conked off into another cat nap.

FREE FAT FREIGHT

The Kefauver Committee ought to know about Elmer's racket. There's no telling how many times he cheated the airlines with his hidden suitcase. The amount of "excess baggage" he smuggled aboard!

The novelty of me wore off soon after the honeymoon. Eating took the place of dancing. Elmer preferred "that piece of pie you saved for me" to "The Waltz You Saved for Me."

In the old days Linda, our daughter, and I could fix Elmer's approximate position in an airplane by the way

My Life with Girth

it listed. Linda could spot her daddy the minute his breadbasket squeaked through the plane's door.

Since he's lost 40 pounds, though, Linda says: "Where's Daddy?"

It used to chafe me no end to have a stranger complain to a friend of mine, "Isn't it terrible the way Beth makes her old father mow the lawn!"

Funny how fat boys always look older than thin ones.

OUR SIZZLE FIZZLED OUT

When I married Elmer the slogan at "Sizzle Ranch," our home, was: "Where the East Peters Out." That was logical, since Fort Worth is advertised as the place "Where the West Begins."

But once Elmer began his "for sure" diet Sizzle Ranch's slogan became: "Where the *Eats* Peter Out."

For a time I passed off Elmer's diet threats as unadulterated fat-boy gibberish. But a grass widow gave him a compliment and I realized this was the real thing.

What a Fat Boy won't do for a grass widow! Especially a redheaded one.

It's a matter of record, as our saggy-springed bathroom scales can tell you, that Elmer slimmed down from 230 to 186 pounds.

My Life with Girth

FAT BOY PSYCHOLOGY FOR WIVES

Girth control has as many angles as birth control. It needs a wife's cooperation.

When your husband gets that remorseful look in his eye, encourage him to diet.

He'll only get as far as the nearest seven-course meal unless you give him moral support.

Kid him. Trick him. Everything goes in the Beltline Sweepstakes.

Don't ignore the old walrus when he waddles home some night and vows he's swearing off the sweet and starchy stuff.

Hide the frying equipment. Bring out the boiler and the broiler.

If he still insists on "just a dab" of fattening foods, spoil them.

A swell way to discourage Starchy Archy is to use vegetable colors indiscriminately.

Unless he's too far gone he'll turn up his nose at pistachio mashed potatoes, for example, or indigo rice.

FEED HIM LIGHT—BUT FAST

Cut his cocktail time to the quick. Before he's finished the first one, give him one to the midriff with a "Dinner's ready."

This rules out an alcoholic appetite.

Then give him a bowl of light soup. It fills him. En-

My Life with Girth

courage a second or third bowl—they only have about 25 calories each.

Load the table with celery, pickles, carrot sticks—any lightweight food to keep his mouth full so he can't clamor for something more substantial.

As his stomach begins to shrink, so will your problem. It takes about seven days to get his stomach back to gentleman size.

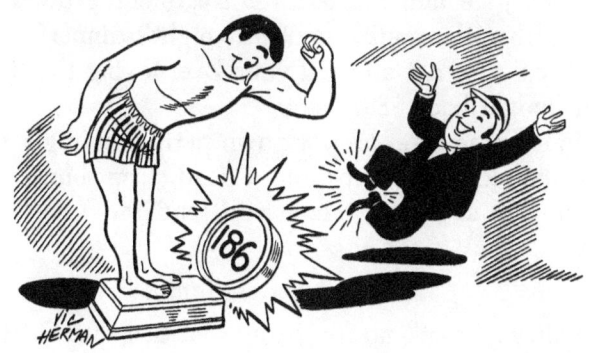

Caution: Never laugh at Mr. Triple Chins. He'll get glum and slink off somewhere to eat a pan of apple dumplings—and you'll be back in the bedroom with a fatso.

SOME DIABOLICAL WIFELY TRICKS

Some well-planned table conversation can have a depressing effect on your chubby hubby's calorie intake.

An operation, for example.

My Life with Girth

How the surgeon just got in there and helped himself. Don't miss a gory detail.

An argument just before dinner is a dandy way to stifle the flow of a fat boy's gastric juices. You're on your own here.

You might start reading the obituary columns. Tell him how a certain banker kicked the bucket at an early age, adding, "He was such a *big* fellow, too."

Then give him the leftover treatment. How a Fat Boy loathes the remnants of last night's dinner!

Buy a new hat and tell your Ever-loving that it set your budget back $80.

In extreme cases, at your own peril, you might wait until the old boy slumps into a dead sleep some night, waken him and say: "Have you read the Kinsey Report?"

TAKE IT FROM ME, GIRLS

Believe me, it's no fun being shackled to a Fat Boy.

His aches, pains, and acute inactivity will wear you down.

Helping the Fat Boy in your life make the fight of his life for an Errol Flynn figure is worth while.

True, you will feel more secure with a chubby hubby—nobody else wants him!

But remember, too: Lean Toms are more tempestuous.

LOVER COME BACK TO ME—*Poor Mrs. Wheeler's Almanac.*

WHAT'S YOUR "HEALTH I.Q."?

You can fight fat with knowledge alone—and eat 3 "squares" a day, and still lose weight. In order to determine your "Health I.Q.," fill in this quiz sheet. Check 1 for highest calorie meal; 2 for next highest; 3 for lowest.

Breakfasts
Which meal has the most—which the least—calories?

Prune Juice	Orange Juice	Tomato Juice
2 Boiled Eggs	Cereal with Milk	1 Fried Egg
2 Slices Whole Wheat	White Toast (1)	Slice of Rye Bread
Coffee Black	Coffee with Sugar	Strawberries—no cream

Lunches

Consomme	Onion Soup	Chicken Broth
Avocado Salad	Coleslaw	Half Head Lettuce
Hot Dog on Bun	Filet	Olives—Celery
Tea with Lemon	Baked Spud (butter)	Sliced Chicken
Orange Ice	Chocolate Ice Cream	Tea with Sugar

Dinners

Fruit Cup	Caviar	Lobster (butter)
Turkey (dark)	Turkey (white)	3 French Fries
Giblet Gravy	Giblet Gravy	Cabbage Salad
Slice Watermelon	Cantaloupe (half)	2 Biscuits
Black Coffee	Slice of Cheddar	Spoon of Honey

NOW CHECK WHICH YOU THINK THE MOST FATTENING

Ripe or Green Olives	Watermelon or Cantaloupe	Orange or Pear
Prune or Orange Juice	Clams or Oysters	Chili or Sliced Ham
Orange Juice or Scotch	Stewed Rhubarb or Pie	Cheese (American) or Caviar

Is This True or False? (Check Answer)

Eating before beltime puts on most weight? ____Yes ____No
Brick ice cream has more calories than handpacked? ____Yes ____No
Water with meals is most fattening? ____Yes ____No

CHECK THE FOLLOWING

1. Which has the most *Vitamin A?* ____Orange Juice? ____Tomato Juice?
2. Which has the most *Vitamin B?* ____Sunshine? ____Oranges? ____Gum Drops?
3. Which has the most *Calcium?* ____Chocolate Bar? ____Watermelon? ____Spinach?
4. Which has the most *Iron?* ____Pork Liver? ____Calf's Liver? ____Jello?

LEARN HOW TO FIGHT FAT WITH KNOWLEDGE
(*Answers on following page*)

ANSWERS TO "HEALTH I.Q."

The first meal in each line has the most calories, the second the next most. The third meal has the least calories of all, even though at times you figure it has the most.

That is where a knowledge of CALORIES helps Fat Boy pick and lose.

Other Answers

Ripe have more calories than green olives.
Prune much more than orange juice.
Orange juice, though, has more than Scotch.
Watermelon far more than cantaloupe.
Clams and oysters are the same—10 each.
Stewed rhubarb 200, most pies 300.
Orange, pear, potato, apple: 100 each.
Chili and sliced ham—the same, 150.
Cheese has 100—caviar just 25!

Did any of these fool you? They didn't fool your calorie countin' tummy!

True or False?

All are "No!" Even having *aqua pura* with meals.

Answers to "Check The Following"

1. Tomato juice—by far!
2. None have B-1—and did that fool you, I bet!
3. Chocolate bar. Bet you figured spinach!
4. Pork. Jello has none. But bet you picked beef!

See how you you can give yourself a Caloric Mickey-Finn by not knowing what's in what you eat?

How to
KILL THE KALORIE IN THE KITCHEN

**To you these secrets I divulge
In winning "The Battle of the Bulge"**

Paste this inside the pantry door. It will help the chief cook and bottle washer kill the kalorie BEFORE it hits FATSO.

BOIL, BROIL AND BAKE
When you do this much of the fat drops into the fire—and not his tummy! (Or your own!)
Besides, it tastes better and you can eat about TWICE as much as of foods that are fried.

WATCH THE INGREDIENTS
Leave out too much lard, butter, oleo and flour in "mixing" of foods.
Side-step too much salt and sugar, and such high-caloric ingredients as nuts, dried fruits and syrups.
In this way you "trap" the Kalorie in the Kitchen!

COOK "SMALL PORTIONS"
Many a fatso hates to "leave good foods behind." He thinks it wasteful, and he is right.
So cook "just enough" to go around **once!** What isn't in front of him can't get down his gullet.

CHOOSE THE RIGHT UTENSILS
Frying pans with humps in the middle, drain off a lot of fat.
There are many such utensils sold today that will drain off excess fat, yet preserve vitamins. Shop around for them.
For example, fried bacon can have 75 calories, but crisped on a "bacon crisper" it has only 25 calories.

Any good cook can use her "thinking cap" in the preparation of foods, to "trap" calories BEFORE they sink Old Fatso at the table. So learn the art of Killing the Kalorie in the Kitchen.

WHEN YOU EAT DON'T CHEAT

THE FAT BOY'S BOOKS
Copyright 1951, 1952 by Elmer Wheeler

www.ingramcontent.com/pod-product-compliance
Lightning Source LLC
LaVergne TN
LVHW011912080426
835508LV00007BA/486